THROUGH MANIC EYES

By Christina Chicklowski Staples

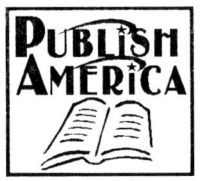

PublishAmerica
Baltimore

© 2009 by Christina Chicklowski Staples.
All rights reserved. No part of this book may be reproduced, stored in a retrieval system or transmitted in any form or by any means without the prior written permission of the publishers, except by a reviewer who may quote brief passages in a review to be printed in a newspaper, magazine or journal.

First printing

PublishAmerica has allowed this work to remain exactly as the author intended, verbatim, without editorial input.

ISBN: 978-1-61582-296-6
PUBLISHED BY PUBLISHAMERICA, LLLP
www.publishamerica.com
Baltimore

Printed in the United States of America

Dedication

This book is dedicated in memory of
my dear friend Jimmy Dempsey
Thank you for all of your support this could have never been
completed without your faith and friendship.

Table of Contents

Page 11-12 Introductory
Page 13-14 Manic Mind
Page 15-16 Symptoms
Page 17-36 My Beginning
Page 37 Jesus Walks Right Next to Me
Page 38-39 A Glimpse into My World
Page 40 Internal Battle
Page 41 Bizarre Thoughts
Page 42-43 Aches of Loneliness
Page 44-46 Lonely Emotions
Page 47-48 Sleepless Nights
Page 49 I Just Don't Fit In

Family & Friends

Page 50 In Honor of My Family & Friends
Page 51 In Loving Memory of Grampy
Page 52-53 Eulogy
Page 54 Grampy's One Year Anniversary
Page 55-56 Grampy's Second Year Anniversary
Page 57 In Honor of Tricia Jacobs
Page 58-59 Tricia's Wedding
Page 60 In Honor of My Wedding
Page 61 Wedding Day
Page 62 In Honor of Kelley Dasso Devantier
Page 63-64 Kelley's Wedding
Page 65 High School Hell
Page 66-67 No Longer Your Best Friend

Depression and Despair

Page 68 Crash Test Dummy
Page 69 My Show
Page 70-72 Worth What It Cost
Page 73-74 My Final Farewell
Page 75-77 Farewell
Page 78-79 Forgive Me
Page 80 No Human on Earth
Page 81-82 The Haunting
Page 83 Here We Go Again
Page 84 Severity of Depression
Page 85-87 Somebody Tell Me Why?
Page 88-89 Stand and Wait
Page 90 Someone
Page 91 Never Belong
Page 92-93 Empty
Page 94-95 A Clearer Vision
Page 96-97 What I Endured to Grow
Page 98-99 How Much More Must I Bleed?
Page 100-101 Scattered
Page 102-103 Disregard
Page 104-105 Hurricane
Page 106-107 Gun
Page 108-109 The War
Page 110-111 Walking for Miles
Page 112-113 Endangered Species
Page 114-115 Tears Keep Falling to the Floor

Rage, Paranoia & Anxiety

Page 116 Enduring Paranoia
Page 117 Rage's Downward Spiral
Page 118 -119 Dream
Page 120-122 Judge a Book by Its Cover
Page 123-124 Who I Am
Page 125-126 Case of Rage
Page 127 Black Hole
Page 128-129 Dying
Page 130-131 Awake
Page 132-133 Too Selfish to Care
Page 134-136 Lonely
Page 137 I Want to Die
Page 138 Ocean
Page 139-140 Overcome You
Page 141-142 Hall of Mirrors
Page 143 God's Wounded Bird
Page 144 Don't Want to Live
Page 145 Thank You
Page 146 The End

Acknowledgements:

To my mother and father who have been the most supportive, loving, and honorable people I have ever encountered. Thank you for all you have done and continue to do. All the good in me comes from your unconditional love and support. I would never take any different even if I could choose. Not all people who are mentally ill have the support that they need and I am so blessed to have you for parents. At my worst you picked me up and found a way to get me through it. There are no words to describe the love I have for you both. There is no way to express the gratitude or appreciation for the life you have given me. Thank you for the thousands of tears you wiped away and the numerous times you picked me up and sent me on my way again. I am so grateful to have you for parents. To Tricia and Joey the best brother and sister any one could ask for. Thank you for all of your love and support and the friendship we share. Tricia, thank you for being my mother hen and always taking care of me. You help me in every thing you do, and you define the true meaning of a sister. Joey growing up we were always so close and you helped me more than you could ever know. You protected me and have given a "big brother" it's true meaning. Not many people can say their brother and sisters are their best friends but I am so thankful for

how close we are. To my husband: you are the best thing that ever happened to me. We had to work hard but it was worth it. Thank you for your unconditional love and support and for caring for me when times are tough. You saved me from a time when I was on a downward spiral and I thank you. I love you and look forward to spending our life together. Some people never find true love in a lifetime, and we have it and live it to the fullest meaning I am so lucky to have you in my life and have all the love even through the worst times you were always there. I love you so much. To Yiayia, you have been the kindest, most giving and loving grandmother a grandchild could ask for. It has been a wonderful, comforting life having you always there. Anything I ever needed I knew I could always count on you. To Theia Sue, Theia Kal, Nick, and Chris having the close family bond we did growing up helped me to be the person I am today I could not ask for a better family. To grandma Pat I have inherited a lot of similarities from you, you were always a wonderful grandmother to us grandkids bringing us places, buying us beautiful gifts, and the memories I have are priceless thank you I love you very much. To Kelley Dasso Devantier and Kristina Kenney Ramos thank you for twenty years of true and loyal friendship I could have never made it without you. Most of the happiest times of my life have been shared with the two of you. To my mother in law Kathy Staples thank you for always being there to listen and talk and always be willing to help in any way that you can. I love you very much and am lucky to have a relationship with you like I have.
To Uncle Charlie, the best uncle I could ever ask for.
And to Heidi Miller thank you for eleven years of support throughout this illness, I could not have survived it without you. To all of my other friends and family that I love so much thank you I would not be the person I am today without all of the shared experiences we have had together. Carrie (Bill) Forgue, Tiffany

Bennet, Liz Chapin, Sarah Booth, my two brother in laws Darren, and Michael, my sister in law Angie, my nephew Julius, just to name a few. And to so many others. If I went on I would go on forever and I love you all very much. You know who you are and I thank you for all you have done. This book could not have been completed without all of the friendship and love I have found in all of you. And special thanks to Yassir Soffan for helping me all those times with my computer, which gave me the ability to complete this book. And also to my two grandfathers Sotirios Vakakas and Joseph Chicklowski. I will miss you and love you forever. And thank you to all who helped make this book possible especially Jimmy Dempsey whose love and encouragement gave me the inspiration for accomplishing this book, I will miss you forever.

My name is Christina Chicklowski Staples.
I am twenty six years old and suffer from bipolar disorder.
I wrote this manuscript in the hope of helping others like me.
This is my story of battling bipolar disorder.
You will endure the daily changes of mood and emotion and catch a glimpse into the world of the bipolar mind.
I have felt that in writing this manuscript I can build awareness,
And show others who suffer from the same disorder that they are not alone.
I have worked for a very long time hoping that one day I can give those like me the strength to keep going.
So this is my story, this is my life.
This is the world of bipolar disorder.

In this book you will encounter a range of emotions. It is a diary of all different stages inside the mind of bipolar disorder. There are days of anger and rage; days of depression and despair; days of hope and positive thinking; and days where I did not want to live.

This range of emotions will give you a glimpse into the life of a manic mind. To see all of the different stages and how the emotions change so rapidly, will give you a better understanding of the daily trials of bipolar disorder. So here is the diary of a manic mind.

Bipolar disorder, or Manic depression is a growing problem. It occurs in about one to two persons out of every hundred. Bipolar is a recurrent affective mood illness characterized by alternating periods of extreme highs and extreme lows.

Bipolar Disorder is a mental illness that occurs in episodes. It can occur in episodes of mania (which are periods of extreme elation and increased mental activity.)

Or attacks of depression (periods of abnormal sadness.) while the causes of Bipolar Disorder are unknown, research shows that some people maybe genetically predisposed to respond readily with manic or depressive episodes due to internal or external influences.

Symptoms of Mania:
*Increased energy, activity, restlessness, racing thoughts, and rapid talking
*Denial that anything is wrong
*Excessive "high" or euphoric feelings
*Extreme irritability and distractibility
*Decreased need for sleep

*Unrealistic beliefs in one's ability and powers
*Uncharacteristically poor judgement
*A sustained period of behavior that is different from the person's usual behavior
*Increased sexual drive
*Abuse of drugs, particularly cocaine, alcohol, and sleeping medication
*Provocative, intrusive, or aggressive behavior
*Paranoia
Symptoms of Depression
*Persistent sad, anxious, or empty moods
*Feelings of hopelessness or pessimism
*Feelings of guilt, worthlessness, or helplessness
*Loss of interest or pleasure in ordinary activities, including sex
*Decreased energy, a feeling of fatigue or being "slowed down"
*Difficulty concentrating, remembering, or making decisions
*Restlessness or irritability
*Sleep disturbances
*Loss of appetite and weight, or weight gain
*Chronic pain or other persistent bodily symptoms that are not caused by physical disease
*Thoughts of death or suicide, including suicide attempts

    People tend to think of mania as being an infectious good mood. But mania is no laughing matter. Most people are irritable and argumentative during their manic episodes.
    There impulsive and impatient and most people just want to duck and get out of the way.
    During manic episodes, the ill may destroy relationships, ruin reputations, or create financial disasters. Doctors also find Bipolar Disorder hard to spot since Bipolar patients rarely complain of manic symptoms. So they are treated for depression instead.

Sometimes I forget how worse things were. How much better I am.

I always carried something as a child very over emotional, extremely sensitive, and very self conscious for being so. I did not like going to school I always missed my Mom and Dad. I would cry and long for my safety net. Where I was always accepted, and always loved, and always secure.

I worried about things a child shouldn't. What if my parents died while I was gone? When my sister and brother were at the same school I felt a little better. They loved me, we were so close.

I remember frequently pulling them out of class crying that I missed Mom.

The detachment was almost heart breaking for me even though it was only hours until I would see them, it felt like years.

I would often be sick with stomach aches probably caused by anxiety. Or maybe I talked myself into it so I could stay home with them. Or one of my grandparents if my parents were at work.

My two best friends lived only a street away and I could not sleep over because when it was time to go to bed I would get anxiety and miss them. For years at sleepover birthday parties I would lie and say I could not spend the night, I could only attend until night time.

As I grew older I remember being sad and since I did not know the reason it remained unexpressed.

Only when it seemed like I had temper tantrums. I am not so sure that's what they always were.

I can remember feeling suicidal in the fifth grade, writing it down how could I tell anyone that?

I remember always feeling sad that my Papoo died. I was only going on four years old when he died, but I remembered him and how much I loved him and that he adored me. I did not understand death but I realized his absence. I can always remember being on family vacations with my parents friends and their kids and just feeling so different. Like I didn't fit in. Like there was something not right with me. Now it all makes sense, but back then it was hard because being a child and not knowing why you felt different, and why you didn't fit in was emotionally draining.

As time went on early teenage years the nightmare started to begin.

At thirteen I cut my arm for the first time. I did not fully understand why. I knew I had a fight with my friends and felt misunderstood I felt rage.

I remember them getting even more mad, and my parents too. My sister and brother seemed to think it was for attention, I am sure it seemed that way.

I didn't get help right away it was only frequent visits to the adjustment councelour at school did they finally send a letter to my parents.

My family sent me to a therapist who I have been with ever since. I loved her finally someone understood me. If it wasn't for Heidi Miller I don't think I would be here today.

I did not start medications until about six months after my first visit. We tried herbal therapies such as St. John's wart. I think it scared my parents to put me on pills at such a young age.

They thought at first that I was clinically depressed they put me on Zoloft. I don't remember it ever helping.

Of course hormones probably made things more difficult to figure out. Adolescence is hard enough without all this added stress.

By this time I was in high school and loving it. I was very social but my grades were declining. When I would come home from school I wanted to sleep not do homework.

Looking back now I am surprised I graduated. My friends started partying young and I was on top of the world, life of the party and loving every minute of it.

It was the only time I had no worries I felt elated. But after drinking was over I would be in worse shape.

I remember fits of rage while getting ready for parties, and at sleepovers, it was starting to take toll on my friendships.

They didn't want to be around depression who could blame them? But it hurt because I was very empathetic and sensitive to others. I had a great gift of walking in other people's shoes, I could feel like they felt just by listening to them.

I overdosed while sleeping over a friends house I honestly don't remember why. Impulse I guess.

When the ambulance came half of the basketball team showed up and saw me being carried out.

I was mortified. I am sure people talked like it was for attention. Maybe it was. I was saying look at me I am in pain! Will you notice now? Will someone please understand? It never worked that way.

Oh kids were so nice calling and visiting. I spent that night in the cardiac care unit after having my stomach pumped, my parents crying. I felt guilty.

Story of my life. Things did not get better. I tried hard to not show it I knew I would lose my friends, eventually I did. But they were never real friends. The real friends are still by my side today. Eventually my doctors started switching medications when their were no signs of improvement.

I became an insomniac. By this time my family was very accepting and trying to help in every way they could. We did family therapy and it helped so much. I can remember my sister petting my head and rubbing my back trying to help me fall asleep. But my brain kept me awake.

The school was aware of what was going on, and they worked out a few arrangements.

I could come into school late if I needed to and would not get detention. Also if I became to sleepy I could take naps in the nurses office.

I took numerous weeks off to do day programs in hospitals.
By senior year I gained thirty pounds if I remember correctly it was when I was on effexor and celexa.

Also by senior year I had two friends that I loved drift away from me. I knew why but it hurt because I couldn't help who I was and I couldn't expect them to stay and help. Some people just are not capable to deal with heavy things. It doesn't mean it didn't hurt because it did.

I felt betrayed because the kind of person that I am I would have stayed by their side.

But not everyone is like me, I learned that lesson over and over.

I remember feeling used after this friend I was extremely close called me out of the blue.(we used to talk ten times a day) but she only wanted me to write her something for a school project. The sad thing was I did it and only out of loyalty. I soon regretted it.

She was getting praised for something I did. But that was just like her to do so.

I lost many friends in high school but mostly out of betrayl on their end.

Deceit is the thing I hate most in the world, I never thought it was hard to be honest.

But this was a different betrayl it just proved what kind of superficial friends they really were.

I am not angry anymore I could care less, some people just do not have it in them it is not my place to judge.

A mutual friend we had all been close to died, we buried him the first day of our senior year.

That depressed me more. That is when empathy and sensitivity become a fault

I had a hard time letting go of this sadness and I became very close to his mother.

She is one of the strongest most inspirational people I ever knew. I loved her very much, we were very close for a long time. We have since lost touch and I only hope that it was because she needed to let go. I think about her often and still love her just as much. I hope if one day she reads this she will know how she touched my life.

By the time senior year was coming to a close I was ready to move on. It was that summer that I met my husband only I did not know it yet.

When we started off neither of us was in a good place, and neither of us wanted anything serious.

As we came to know each other though I thought he was wonderful. He was so different he did not turn away from me because I was depressed. Even in my rages he did not turn away. He was sensitive to me.

That made me fall in love. All other boyfriends thought I was weird for having cuts on my arms, and going from laughing to sad to rage in the matter of moments.

Not Teddy he loved me anyway.

I was seventeen when we started dating and those first years were not always good.

But when I look back now we saved each other.

So before I get ahead of myself let me get back to that summer.

We were having fun anticipating college in the fall.

When it came it was not all it was cracked up to be.

When I started their were lots of kids from high school their.

I was in the local community college. College was so different it was all up to you very laid back in comparison to high school. The fact that I could skip classes and not get detention didn't help. If I was too tired or depressed I would not get in trouble if I didn't go. So I didn't. I made it through about three months.

It was hard for me I was taking the same courses that I was in high school, only they backed me up to pre-algebra, I took that freshman year. It was depressing I didn't know what I wanted to do and even when I did it would take me forever to accomplish it. I had friends say anything I started I never finished. They were right, only they probably thought it was because of something else not the illness, if they even recognized that I had an illness.

I didn't handle stress well at all, no one does but I couldn't even function. I was the only one in my family who would not complete college that was hard to swallow I felt even more different.

So I took a break from college and enjoyed being with my friends, I wanted to work too.

When I couldn't make it through working part time either my mom decided it was time we do something.

She was paying hundreds of dollars a month in prescriptions and doctors for me and supporting me.

We were told that I should try applying for disability it would help for the prescriptions mostly.

Some people get denied over and over and it takes years for them to get it, some never do.

I received approval within a month, I guess it goes to show those who thought it was an attention game that my medical files stated that their was a significant problem.

I overdosed again after getting in a fight with my father, it was impulse and rage, I regretted this time more than any mistake I ever made in my life.

They did not pump my stomach they made me drink charcoal. It was like drinking car oil.

I have never been so violently ill in all of my life. I immediately had diarrhea and began vomiting I did not stop for two days. I remember my mothers taunting voice "are you ever going to do this again?" I haven't since. The doctor finally prescribed a suppository to relieve nausea and vomiting, I have never been so grateful in all my life. I also knew I did not want to die. Sometimes I did only so I would not have to feel the way I did. The prospect of not having to think or feel was tantalizing. But I knew how it would hurt my family and being religious I knew it was not my choice, I just had to keep going there is no other choice.

I know why people kill themselves, I know why I tried. This illness is very lonely and people do not understand. You can say I am bipolar and it is just a statement to many.

They only see the side where you appear like any one else.

When a person has cancer you can see the illness,

When a person is mentally ill it is internal it is not visible. Maybe when you act out but then it is thought of as weird or for attention.

So when I did not return to college things became pretty bad.

Most of my other friends were moving on with their lives. I was hanging out with a crowd that at the time were not moving ahead they were just partying in the moment. That was okay with me the future seemed overwhelming. But not all of those people were good for me. They liked the fact that I was so giving they abused it, they abused me. My two best friends were drifting away, one went off to college, the other concentrating on her relationship. I understood but I felt extremely lonely. So I clung to these unhealthy people. My own relationship was hard we were not even twenty one so we hung out with our friends, separately a lot so it was so hard to trust one another. It was even harder when twenty one hit. We were so young it's amazing to me that we lasted.

Their were friends I made in that group that were healthy and did last and were still close, the unhealthy ones drifted down their own path. At that time I was changing medications rapidly. Nothing seemed to work and the doctors didn't really know what to do. I suffered immensely. No one around me was going through anything similar and I felt so lonely. It was the time when I was on paxil that things really hit the fan.

I was sick and crying all the time it sent me into a manic phase. My mother cried all the time, I was having fits of rage. I punched through windows, broke her pictures, and a lot of her belongings. The things I could replace I did. I said things to her I would never ever in a million years to her that still to this day make me cry tears of guilt. The rage was so extreme it would come out of no where and it was so strong I felt their was no control. After the anger was out I would lay on the floor and cry my heart out. And after all the hurt I would cause my mother she would still come comfort me because she could not bear to hear me cry.

The guilt after the rage was so extreme. At the time I was on paxil I went so manic I beat up a girl something I wouldn't usually do but it was rage. She tried to dance with my boyfriend and it made me flip my lid. I acted out like a crazy person in front of so many people. They seemed to get a kick out of my heartache. After I was in the fight my friend was mad at me for fighting at her house it made me so much more depressed. I knew something was very wrong with me.

The next day after the fight my father brought me to the doctors and as we sat their I was banging my head up against the wall, the doctor looked at my father and said I am sorry I don't know what do with her. They checked me into the hospital that night. I was plagued by paranoid and obsessive thoughts that caused me and my boyfriend to argue constantly. We were so young and immature at the time and I expected him to want to take care of me, but his biggest concern was hanging out with his friends and having fun.

I heard rumors that caused rage and obsessive thinking it hurt so much because I believed my own thoughts, my own scenarios I thought they were reality. It was my councelor that helped me realize that I sometimes had delusional thinking. At this point I was being checked into the hospital I was extremely overweight and depressed about that as well. When people looked at me I was certain they were thinking that I was disgusting. Maybe they were maybe they weren't but I thought they were. I always thought people were talking about me. I trusted no one not even any of my friends.

In the hospital I was sad to be their but it was almost a relief, these people would accept me.

I almost felt more comfortable their than I did at my own home. These people were similar to me.

I worried constantly about what my boyfriend was doing, even though he came to see me.

every time my visitors would leave I would watch them through the window and long to be normal.

It broke my heart every time someone left me. This was one of the lowest points of my life, the loneliest too. I felt abandoned and disconnected from everyone. No one understood me or took the time, they just did not care enough. This was when I came to the realization that I was extremely different from everyone I knew. I felt like everyone left me for dead. Everyone. They were to busy having fun while I was in the depths of despair. I would have given them the support I could, but no one would give me that back. It was the biggest betrayl I ever faced. I still have anger and resentment, and it hurts to remember that people I loved turned there back on me in my darkest hour. I have since accepted it that they may never care, and probably never understand. I knew as a child I did not fit in, but this time in my life was when I had to accept the inevitable. It wasn't easy, but it has since become easier. That was my first and only overnight.

Their was one time before in high school that I was supposed to. But the place was dumpy and I was ever so grateful when my father said "I am not leaving my daughter here." the fact of the matter is no matter how comfortable I was I wanted to be home. I think everyone thought that my hospital stay was going to be a miracle cure but it wasn't .

While I was their the doctors were sympathetic to my weight gain and put me on topomax.

It was like a miracle I lost seventy ponds in about eight months.

I took a creative writing class at school that fall and I noticed that I couldn't even write anymore.

The topomax caused something called cognitive dullness. I would go out with my friends and not even speak. I couldn't even think of anything to say. I was paranoid when I went out to the bars I thought everyone was talking about me and that they thought I was just a tag along. I eventually came off of the topomax when my boyfriend became frustrated that I could not even concentrate enough to drive. I remember him saying you seem so slow, what happened to my girlfriend?

So I was taken off of it. Over the course of three years I gained all the weight back. Still changing medications due to side effects, but I couldn't lose the weight. All the meds I was on caused weight gain, story of my life.

It's funny that these medications used for "depression" cause weight gain, I am always depressed about my weight. Because I know why I am overweight. It almost feels like I am being punished for having this illness.

Things were still pretty bad, I wasn't working or going to school my mother would wake me up in the morning before she went to work, feed me my pills and I would go back to sleep My mother prayed to her father to find some help for me. He answered it by letting her find Massachusetts general hospital. The first time I went their my mom and my sister accompanied me. I had a wonderful doctor she helped me immensely. I started to function again.

Finally I was able to go to school for one class a semester, and work at a convience store as a lottery girl.

That job overwhelmed me.

After awhile I had to take a leave of absence when I began hurting myself again. But when I felt well enough I started back up. Even though I hated the job I stuck with it.

I felt I didn't fit in with anyone, it was very lonely. I wanted to be someone. I wanted an honorable job, that I could feel proud of. But it would take me time to get their. My first doctor in Boston left after two years she appointed me to someone new. But the new doctor I had in Boston around this time who I felt didn't like me that much sent me for psychological testing It lasted six hours. She wanted me to do something called a DBT group. Around this time I was kind of in denial of the illness, because I sometimes felt good.

She seemed to think I had borderline personality disorder and that I was manipulative. She convinced me into getting off my medications to see if I really needed them.

I had recently broken my shoulder and was out of work again I was depressed. I was going out drinking all the time. The night I hit a telephone pole was no exception. I met up with my boyfriend after the clubs let out, and seeing that we were both drunk as usual we fought. We always fought when we both drank. I had terrible reactions to drinking. At first I would be bubbly and having the time of my life. But then I would usually get paranoid and delusional, emotional, and depressed. And depressed for days afterwards.

I also had a fight with his mother that night. I drove around crying hysterically. I don't remember exactly how it happened one minute I was driving looking for my phone the next I was in a telephone pole.

I woke up and could remember thinking "my face is burning"

then I passed out and the next thing I knew I was being pulled out of my smoking car.

The girl that pulled me out called my father and he came over right away. He knew I had drank that night.

It was just like him to protect me. I signed a release form so I did not have to ride in an ambulance.

My father brought me to the E.R.

When I was called in they put me in a neck brace and ordered cat scans and x-rays. I was not in good shape.

I had burns and bruises and a concussion and whip lash. I hurt everywhere. I knew things could have been a lot worse, I could have killed myself, or even worse someone else.

In all the time I was off meds I purposely tried to drive into a tree, tried to cut my wrists with a butcher knife (if it had not been for my brother I would have succeeded) and accidently drove into a telephone pole.

Not to mention the countless tears or rage attacks.

I had lost weight, but it was time to get back on the meds. When I was a little more stable I was hired through a temp agency to work for the gas company. I felt like I was on my way.

The only problem was I had post traumatic concussion syndrome and had trouble remembering new information. I totally failed at my training and they let me go.

I went home and cried on the floor in my mothers arms. It felt like because of this illness I couldn't accomplish even the simplest things. Well simple to the average person but of course life wasn't even manageable for me.

My boyfriend and I decided we both needed change. I decided to go to a dental assisting school in Worcester while he went to a local truck driving school. As hard as it was for me I accomplished it and so did he. One thing I will never forget that he did for me was on my first day of dental school. I was so nervous about making the hour and a half drive by myself that he drove me and waited two hours in the car while I had my first class. But I did the same for him. I was the only one with a car. We shared it. We pretty much went everywhere together so he just saw another car as an unneeded expense. The only problem was his truck driving job was a half hour away and he had to be their for three o'clock in the morning. So I would get up and drive him a half hour their and home in the middle of the night. Even when I was working. But I loved him. Sun, rain, or snow I did it. I never told many people they would talk bad about him letting me do that. Maybe they were just jealous of the love we had for each other I don't know nor do I care.

The bottom line was we stuck together through the worst and helped each other succeed. The dental school accomplishment was huge for me. It wasn't that long ago that I was in bed everyday being fed my medications. It took me a long time to find a job, but when I did it was perfect. The job sort of found me and it was like it was meant for me. A dentist who was working part time and was looking for a part time assistant.

His current assistant was leaving to become a dental hygienist and worked with a girl I went to high school with at another job she had. She told her I was just out of school and was looking for a job, and that I was a good person. She called me and I was called in for an interview. It went great. That week me and Teddy decided to go look at rings to just price them. While we were looking we found one he could afford he asked me if I wanted it. He did not have to ask me twice. I was never so happy in all of my life. That week was the best week in my whole life. I was engaged and was offered the job. All those years of suffering and God answered all of my prayers and changed my life in one week. I fought so hard and had come so far.

I felt alive again. Something worth living for. We decided the wedding would be in two years, so we could save money and get ahead of the game. We never really did get ahead of the game. In august of 2006 one of my husbands best friends was killed on his motorcycle. It was devastating. It also caused my husband to take a huge step back. But who could blame him. He was the happiest most stress free guy it wasn't fair that he died. Well it's never fair that someone dies, but he died way too young and it devastated everyone. As time moves on you learn to live with the pain and grief and things did get easier. That was until November. That's when Grampy fell. Growing up we always had an extremely close family. On my moms side were her two sisters who were like two other mom's and my two boy cousins. We were extremely close with my cousins all growing up their were only five grandkids on mom's side. Yiaya was the only grandparent left because as I said Papoo died when I was very young. And Yiaya is the most wonderful grandparent you could ask for. She would do anything for her grandchildren. She bought me my first car, my wedding dress, my veil, my shoes. She is the most giving, loving grandmother you could ever ask for. On dad's side we had gram's and gramps and dad has a sister and three brothers. We were extremely close to grandma and grandpa. Especially grandpa. He was the kind of Grandpa that was always there to baby sit or just come over to visit with the family. He was always there. Disney world trips, red sox games, and just regular days, he was always there. After he retired grandma and grandpa would go to Florida for the winter after the holidays. Sometimes it feels like he is still just in Florida. I am getting ahead of myself let me get back to November. Grandpa was eighty two he was starting to develop dementia. He had a terrible heart. He had a massive heart attack at the age of fifty three and only had one third of a heart that functioned. He was very religious and the kind of man that would give you the shirt off his back. He loved his family, he was a hard worker, he loved my father. He also had a special connection with my sister. Grandpa had one wish, he never wanted to go into a nursing home and my father made sure he would never see the insides of one. When Grampy started with the dementia family wanted to put him in one but my father would not have it. Now my sister had been sickly through her youth and went to school half days. Grampy would pick her up everyday from school and stay with her, that's the kind of grandfather he was. My sister also had a dream, she had been saying since she was nine that she was going to be a lawyer. My brother and I were like okay (we had no idea what a lawyer was). And grampy always stood behind her dream. But as you get older you get involved in your own life so much and it seemed that Grampy was put on the back burner a little by all of us. I know that is a normal part of life but you suffer for the guilt of it now. You wish you took more time like you did when your own life didn't have so much importance. I will never forget going over to show Grandma and Grandpa my engagement ring. Grampy's eyes were bad and he couldn't see well, but with teary eyes and his sweet voice he said (I can't see it, but it feels beautiful) that memory brings tears to my eyes. So in November of 2006 my sister was finished with law school and struggling to pass the bar exam. She was waiting to hear back from the test results that week. That week Dad had his brother move into Grampy's house to help take care of him. But the night before he did Grampy got up to use the bathroom in the middle of the night, he slipped in the bathroom and hit his head.

They brought him to the emergency room and he seemed okay so they brought him home, little did we know he was not okay. My sister learned she passed the bar exam we were so proud of her, I remember I brought her a dozen roses. The next day she went to tell Grampy but he was sleeping. I will never forget that Sunday Mom, Dad, and I were in the living room when Dad received a call from Uncle Charlie (Grandma's brother) that something was not right with Grandpa. We decided to go over there. I suggested that we call Tricia. When we went over their the sight I saw will be etched in my memory forever.

They had a mattress on the living room floor and Grampy frail in his pajamas was laying there having convulsions, they had mittens on his hands so he would not scratch his face. I immediately started sobbing. I knew from that moment that he was going to die. I was running around crying as we waited for the ambulance and I will never forget my sister saying to me go home your not strong like me and Dad. You can't handle this. You see everyone always protected me, because of the illness they never wanted me to have any extra stress. She was just trying to protect me, but I would later prove to be stronger than they thought. Grampy blamed himself for my illness it ran on his side of the family and when it worsened for me he would cry and tell me he was sorry. Being as religious as he was he would say I pray for you everyday, and I know he did. It wasn't his fault I was sick it's just the luck of the draw. Well they admitted Grampy into the hospital again he had fluid in his brain, they said he only had ten percent of his brain functioning .

I remember calling my Mom from work to see how he was and asking her if she thought he would be okay.

She said it doesn't look good I think you need to go see him. I went after work that day. I can remember what uniform I wore every detail of that time. When I arrived at the hospital I brought a prayer book with me. I was alone (we all came at different times due to work). I figured I could pray for him seeing as he couldn't. I can remember rubbing his head and kissing his cheek as he lay there I knew he was dieing and as I prayed for him holding his hand my heart broke. I began to sob. And as I sobbed he opened his eyes and sat up staring at me clearly visibly upset by my tears.

I stopped crying, shocked. He was supposed to only have ten percent of his brain working yet he knew I was there and in pain. I rubbed his hand and kept saying Grampy I am okay I am just upset because your hurting I am okay. I said this until he lay back down still staring at me, I stopped crying and then he closed his eyes again. Here he was dieing and still concerned about me. I went to the hospital everyday until the family made a decision about what to do. The doctors said he would need a feeding tube and have to be in a nursing home or we could take him off of everything and bring him home to die. Knowing his father's wish about never being put in a nursing home my father was forced to make the hardest decision of his life. He was going to bring Grampy home to die.

After Grandpa's discomfort of hearing me cry it gave me great strength. Everyone else was falling apart while I remained composed. We brought him home the Friday before Thanksgiving. We were their every day for eight hours at a time some days but it would feel like only an hour. We would just sit by his bedside holding his hand talking about old memories blessing him with holy water. Seeing as I only worked part time the day before Thanksgiving I was their alone with Grampy. I stayed all day but he would stop breathing for almost a minute at a time and I was growing scared that he would die just the two of us and I would not know what to do. After spending about nine hours there I went home, but that night I could not go back, I was drained. The next day Thanksgiving day we went and stayed until about two thirty we were going to eat something and then go back immediately after. We said good bye and left. Just as we were about to eat my sister called my uncle to tell him the food was ready when he said he thought Grandpa had just passed. We drove their right away. My sister had not even stopped the car and I was running in the house. We laugh now saying Mom, Tricia and I were like a heard of wild buffalo running in the house.

Grandpa was gone it was three o'clock the hour Christ died. (ironic seeing Grampy was such a strong believer in Jesus.) I had to make the hardest phone call, I had to call my father and tell him his Dad was gone. We waited for Hospice to arrive to pronounce him dead. Then we waited for the funeral home to pick him up. My father always told me when I lost friends at young ages (Jesus said he will come like a thief in the night) when the funeral home arrived it was dark and rainy they were in black rain coats and as they wheeled our beloved Grampy out in a body bag they felt like the thieves in the night.

The wake and funeral came and went but the love I have is so strong for him in my heart. Death can not take that away. It's funny how you take the little things for granted, you never realized how important just his prescence was. Even if you weren't sitting there having a conversation with him just seeing him. He was always there growing up and now he's gone. You always know how much you love someone but not being able to tell them and hug them makes you love and cherish them so much more. I will miss his prescense forever. After Christmas time seemed to fly by and my wedding was upon me. My wedding was the happiest day of my life. I was marrying a wonderful loving man who stuck by me in my worst. He loves me honors me and protects me. My parents gave me the most perfect and wonderful wedding. It was just like them to do so. Then they gave us their time share week to take our honeymoon in Aruba. Everything was perfect. We had the most wonderful time in all of my life. We were blessed with a sign of a good marriage my husband won sixty five hundred dollars at a casino their. When we came home things were not so good. My gynecologists office had put me on a new birth control and I was a wreck. I asked them to change it because of severe PMS. What they put me on made it a hundred times worse. I was so emotional. I cried at everything, the drop of a hat.

THROUGH MANIC EYES

The news, our dog we recently took in was way too much of a responsibility for me, but I loved him. The doctors office told me to go see a psychiatrist when I told them what was going on. They were failing me, they were the experts on birth control. My rage was out of control. Here it was the first months we were living together and I was out of my mind. But my husband stood by me although it affected him deeply. I feel for the mentally ill who do not have any support, that has to make the illness so much lonelier and harder to manage. Finally my father put in a call to his friend who is a gynecologist and he did him a favor by seeing me and switching me to a different birth control. It took awhile but it got better. In my battle with this illness I have been on Zoloft, Celexa, Effexor, Riddalin, Ativan, Lithium, Welbutrin, Zonegran, Tegretol, Cymbalta, Clonodine, Seroquel, Geodon, Risperdal, Topomax, Paxil, and Trazadone. I also know their have been more I just cannot remember. I tried and failed on all due to side affects ranging from severe weight gain, to panic, to manic phases, to severe fatigue and cognitive dullness. It has been an unending battle for stability. And now I find myself here. I had cut myself during a rage episode and I knew I needed help. Things were bad again I needed medication changes again and I recently completed another day program in the hospital. I am on another new medication and although my rage has subsided I still have severe anxiety, and have periods in which I go without sleeping I am managing. Things are better right now and I like that. You see to me all of these trials have made me stronger and although there are so many days I want to give up this battle with this illness I don't. and although I still have many struggles (I hardly attend any type of functions. Weddings, funerals, parties, because I never feel good and I never know day to day what my mood is going to be like.) I am taking, Topomax again (an extremely low dose), Trazadone, lamictal, abilify, klonopin, and yaz. I don't feel good half the time and working can be a struggle, but I am living. I am not letting this illness run my life anymore. I am accepting it, understanding it, and learning to live with it. It can be done. I am living proof. So for all of you out there in the same boat who know this road all too well know that you can do it to. There is such a thing as hope. And maybe that is hard to only have hope to cling to and only have hope to keep you going, but at least it's something. And to know that even if you do not know them personally there are people out there who feel the exact same way you do, I am one of them.

So keep doing what you are doing put one foot in front of the other. So the last message I send to all of my friends: when the burden is too heavy, and help seems unknown, I too know your pain, you are never alone.

When you feel no hope, like you cannot get by, keep on going hold your head high. We have been given a trial a roller caster ride, but we must stick together side by side. And although we have not met it has been my privealage to say that I am standing with you struggling through each day.

God wanted me to have this, so I must endure, to have my place in paradise, to walk through heaven's door. I know that we are close, Jesus and I, I am close within his heart, I will be rewarded when I die. I have to try not to be angry let his peace flood through my soul, I will have to trust him and practice self control. People say I am weird but I am special to our lord, I have to deal with pain and sorrow, these things must be endured. No one feels my heart ache not a soul can see, but Jesus knows my pain and walks right next to me. Although in this earthly life I am misunderstood, this I did not ask for, nor is it something that I would. I walk life's path alone with no mortals by my side, but Jesus takes my hand and rewards me for what I have been denied. Yes I have this illness but god has bigger plans, he has given me a gift and beside me is where he stands. Yes my loved ones feel annoyed because they do not get my pain, I will try to forgive them, it is something they cannot contain. So I feel disconnected from this life, in this darkness light has shown, because Jesus walks right next to me so I will never be alone.

I always knew something was wrong. When people told me to snap out of it, and I couldn't. I lived in another world, but that world was my mind. As a child I was sad, extremely sensitive, with no reason to be. I felt guilty, like I had no right to feel as I did.

I kept my feelings hidden so I would not hurt anybody. But I was dying inside.

I was always oversensitive, sensitive to a fault I say now. When I cried I felt I couldn't stop, I could cry for hours. I was so emotional I felt that I was feeling the whole world's sadness. Why did I feel emotional when I would see someone different? Someone mentally challenged would make me cry for the pain and judgement they would endure. I felt it so strongly like it was me enduring it.

Maybe I felt the pain because I was different too, and I couldn't help it either.

Maybe all of us who don't fit the "normal criteria" of today's society feel each other's pain? I am not sure all I know is that I feel everything to an intensity that I myself do not understand. Sometimes I wonder does everyone think like me? Is everyone in pain?

Does everyone think about the same things over and over again until they believe their own conclusions are reality? And try to figure out am I manifesting this or is it real?

Try to admit that. Could someone make a comment to you and you analyze it obsess about it and then believe your own conclusions because that's what feels right?

Can others sleep without meds? Or do they also not sleep without them because their brain can not stop racing about everything and anything?

Is everyone sad for at least two weeks out of every month for no apparent reason?

I wonder what it is like to be normal? What is normal? Certainly not me. Otherwise I wouldn't feel so lonely. I have only known myself, how I work. I remember coming to the sad conclusion that my friends did not think or feel what I did, it was hard accepting that others did not care as much as I did. That they did not have the emotional capacity that I did. Something that would affect me would not affect them the same.

I know that at one point while I was in the hospital, with others like me, for that brief time, I felt I did belong. I felt more comfortable with people that were like me.

Almost as comfortable as you feel with your own family.

But I am no longer ashamed, I am no longer going to hide my illness, I have finally accepted it enough to put it out their for the world to see. So here I am. The real me, all the struggles, secrets, and a glimpse into the soul of a mentally ill person who is no longer afraid of what the world will think.

So here it is another day. My only way to cope and express is through this page.

Why? Because I can't call up my friends and say "hey I thought that this guy could read my thoughts, and that my phone was transmitting messages without me helping it or me wanting it to." No that's not a joke. Those are some real thoughts. Paranoid ones that I deal with. Then I have to work it out and convince myself that it's not really that way just how I perceive it. No I am not being followed, no one is mad at me. I have to keep it bottled up inside because the world does not understand it. I don't understand it, want it, or like it. There are days I don't want to leave the house. I have this act down so well that no one has a clue that anything is wrong. But while I talk to you there is an internal battle that is being fought, and I am not sure how much longer I am going to have the strength and the will to keep fighting.

Today is a day I want to give up, but I have to take my own advice and keep going.
There has to be someone out there in this world that is like me. I wish I didn't feel so alone.
I hate when people ask me why I am sad. What doesn't make me sad is a better question.
My sensitivity is more like a curse then a quality. I get sad from commercials, the news, things that have not happened yet. Things I can't control. Sometimes I sit here and wonder is this real? Am I real? Sometimes I feel like I am not in tune with reality, or maybe I am so in tune with reality and everyone else is weird. I am normal because everything makes me cry, and I feel like I cannot stop. I hate change. It seems that I cannot deal with everyday life people die everyday, people work everyday, people are sick, they have to pay bills and do housework, so why do I feel like crawling in a hole and dieing from almost all of those things? I wish I did not have to feel, because everything hurts and it is lonely because if I express bizarre thoughts to the people I know they would look at me different.

Do you ever wish you could go back to being a child? I find myself wishing for it a lot.

When I was a child I still remember being sad and misunderstood, overly sensitive, but my family loved me accepted me, and adored me, so it was okay to be different, because they loved me anyway.

As I have grown older it is harder to feel accepted, I know I am different, I do not think and feel things the way everyone else does. I am called weird for something I have no control of. It amazes me that I can be surrounded by people and still feel the ache of loneliness . It is frustrating when you are trying to understand yourself and you feel like you are being attacked because of who you are. What I mean by being attacked is mood swings tend to be mistaken as being a bitch, and paranoia is thought of as weird, and your tears are annoying, and your depression is draining, and your fatigue is typical.

It is not easy trying to be who you are when most people do not understand, or care to understand or maybe do not have it in them to understand.

I want to be happy and be who they want me to be, it hurts me more than it hurts them, I do not enjoy waking up everyday not knowing is it going to be a good day? Or one I am going to have to struggle through.

People do not try to get it they think you have the power to stop it, but why would I go through this torture if I did not have to. But the fact of the matter is you could never get it unless you have endured it. I am not feeling sorry for myself, this is the only way to express myself, without being judged. It is a difficult cross to bear, especially since it is overlooked by many as an illness. But an illness it is indeed, with no cure. Medications are tough, I have been on most. The heart wrenching part is the realization that there are no more options, and that acceptance may be the most lonely part of this disease. I do not want to waste my life drowning in this disease, I want to live it to the fullest. I do not want to hurt anymore, or hurt the people that I love. For all the people out there who know this ache, keep going, keep trudging through on the hope that one day things will get better. It is a long road to happy maybe one day we will get there too.

After all, In a way I can not be annoyed that they do not try to understand, after all who wants to know the aches of loneliness? I know I don't. But what may I ask is happy? I hope one day to find that answer and hold it in my heart for all the days of my life.

In my poems I talk of being alone. In life I have people around me that I love and are supportive, but what I mean by saying alone is the people I love and people I know do not understand me they do not think the way I think. They do not feel things to the intensity that I do. That is fine with me I would not wish people to have the mind I do. It is hard to feel connected when you know they cannot relate to you. Everyone is different. Every person is sad at some point in their lives. That I can relate to. It has been hard to accept that I am sad just because. I wish I knew why my brain does not work "properly." I wish I had a fix it solution. It would make my life and my families lives much easier. But this journey I endure has been hard to accept but I am accepting it now. Other people in the world feel how I do, maybe not people I know, but people out there do. I feel that if I can write how I feel then the people out there who experience the same things can also know that there are people out there who know exactly what they are going through.

    It is hard I understand myself even if people around me do not. I can laugh now at my rage. What other person that I know has a rage attack if the dog pees on the floor? Not anyone I am connected to. And I have a puppy and he has accidents a lot I do not freak out every time he has an accident. So why do I sometimes? Why is it I can be in a great mood and some unwanted thoughts pop into my head and it changes me completely? Why do I get crazy emotions over common things? Well I have a mood disorder is how I explain it to myself. But that does not explain itself to other people. It is just a statement. Some probably think of it as excuses for no self control. But when the emotions take over there is no self control.

I get feelings so intense that I do not know how to vent it. I used to cut my arms simply because I did not know what to do with my anger. Now because it hurts my husband I try to vent it in other ways breaking things, screaming things that I will not even remember later. It is so overwhelming that I always think of hurting myself. But I have improved. I can remind myself that the rage will pass and that helps me not to do things that I will regret. It is hard I am recently married and when I get like this it takes a toll on my husband. I try to tell him when I am feeling "good" not to take it personal. But he is human and I know it hurts. That is when I know it is a selfish disease. Because when I am caught up in these emotions I am only thinking of myself and hating him and everyone else for not understanding. It is not fair to him or me. I do not think if the situations were reversed that I could handle what I put him through. I feel regret as soon as I come down from my rage. I cry misunderstood tears, guilt tears, sorry for myself tears.

It is weird how I hang on negative memories instead of positive ones. It is strange how I feel agitation for no apparent reason, and expect others to feel empathetic. Maybe that is how I am able to be empathetic. Because I long for people to get how I feel. My family especially my mother {God bless her} has been taking care of me for so long that she does not take my abuse to heart. I know it hurts her because she has to put her life on hold to care for me, and ignores her own needs, to make my life more manageable for me. I know I am lucky because it was very hard for me in the beginning because they did not know what to think of me. It might go away. We kept it hidden for awhile. Part of why I can function the way I do is because they accepted me and loved me anyway. There are people out there who would not accept my behavior if I were there child. And I feel for the people who are like me and turned away by their loved ones. It makes this disease even harder and even lonelier.

Sometimes I still can't sleep even though I take my meds. I am aware of being awake thinking of everything and anything. I obsess all night about strange things over and over. I know most people do this at one time or another, but if I do not take something to sleep it would be like this every night of my life. I find it strange that I could stay wide awake for days. How is that possible? I know that it's my brain, but I just don't understand what went wrong.

How could my mother tell me I was the happiest baby and then have this lot in life for being sad? I just don't know I guess it is just one of those mysteries of life, I just wish there were more answers and research on the brain to answer these questions. I find it amazing that man can send men to the moon but they have not figured out the brain yet. I mean we all have brains, they get us through everyday life. So why is it so hard for people to understand that it is possible for the brain to not function the way it is supposed to. I mean with computers you get glitches and viruses, your body gets the flu and diseases, so why is it so hard to accept that the brain can malfunction too? Please keep that in mind while reading this book. There is no such thing as perfect no matter how hard man strives for it. Thank you for your support in purchasing this book and for being interested enough in the daily struggles of the bipolar mind.

So here I am again today,
With a rage explosion to get in my way.
I acted out in front of them again,
It's a place I haven't been.
I haven't been there for some time,
I committed another crime.
Crime of anger, crime of abuse,
Not like I wanted to, it's not like I choose.
I try to tell them, I try to explain,
They just don't get it, they don't know my pain.
I shouldn't have left the house, I was in a delicate state,
And the alcohol helped in sealing my fate.
They say but you were happy, you were fine,
But they do not know the depths of your mind.
They don't see the anxiety, the paranoia nagging,
They don't feel the fatigue, how you are dragging.
They only see the pretty picture, the laughs and the smiles,
While inside your hurting, they don't see how it piles.
It piles up until it overflows, the depth of your heartache nobody knows.
Then when you act out they catch a glimpse,
But they could never get it, those we call wimps.
Don't have the compassion, don't have the brains,
To understand a disorder and what it contains.
I am so different, I feel so alone,
I feel so much guilt, but that can't be known.
Why was I made this way? I do not like it at all.
I never had a choice, god made the call.
And it's so unfair, it breaks my heart in two,
This is one of those days I don't know how to make it through.
I can't turn back time, can't reverse the clock.
So here I go again to take this lonesome walk.
The walk where I realize that I am different that I can never win,
This walk where I realize again that I just don't fit in.

I felt it was important to add in a section of family and friends. The reason being, they are extremely important in my life. I look to my family for the support in helping me cope with bipolar disorder. We have always been an extremely close family. My husband jokes and calls us the "Brady Bunch." All I know is that I am lucky and grateful, and that they deserve to be honored in this book.

This poem was written for my Grampy who died on Thanksgiving day of 2006. I know how lucky I was to have him for twenty three years but he impacted my life so much, it is funny you do not realize it until they are gone. This poem is my dedication for everything he did, thank you Grampy You helped make me who I am today. Thanks for the little things, they equal out to all the big things. Thank you I will miss you forever.

IN LOVING MEMORY OF JOSEPH ANTHONY
CHICKLOWSKI
"GRAMPY"
MARCH 20TH, 1924–
NOVEMBER 23,RD, 2006

IN MEMORY OF GRAMPY

When I came to see you I know you heard,
Although you could not speak a word,
I saw it in your eyes you were telling me not to cry,
And I told you it was okay if you had to say good-bye.
I did not want you to be in pain, and I know you were not alone as you walked down Heavens Lane.
Although people say it's life that we all have to die,
It still does not ease the pain, or stop the tears I cry.
When I think of you I think kind, gentle, and warm,
And I know you will still be with us, just not in earthly form.
I wish their was something we could have done different so you would not have to leave, but I know you would not want us to dwell, and hurt, and grieve,
I guess there is no point in thinking what should have been, I know this parting is only temporary, we will all be together again.
There are a few things I want you to know, things that were not said before you had to go.
For you we will try to be strong, Joey your namesake will carry your name on. Tricia your girl passed the bar, I know you're filled with pride where ever you are.
I just wanted to thank you for your prayers everyday,
I don't want you to worry because I will be okay.
I know life is not always fair, it's just on my wedding day I wanted you there.
I know you will still look down with tears and a smile,
And I know you will be with us when daddy walks me down the aisle.
I have so many good memories, too many to write, like how on the weekends you would watch us on mom's bingo night.
I remember sausage grinders and Heinekens at the Sox game, without you life will never be the same.

You were such a good man you gave all you had,
You were a wonderful husband, grandpa, and dad.
I am so sorry for your suffering now it will cease,
And you can find comfort in Heaven's peace.
I knew you would not live forever but how does one prepare? I guess I just brushed it off because you were always there.
And now that the time is here I do not want to say good bye, this doesn't seem real, I wish it was a lie.
I guess I am just oblivious I never thought about this day, And I know that I am selfish, because I wanted you to stay.
My heart is so heavy, I feel so sad, you have been the best grandpa a kid could have had.
I just want you to know that I love you so much, everyone loves you, do you see the lives you touch?
In life you never know what awaits, but I know I don't have to worry Grampy, because you have entered Heavens Golden Gates.

FOR "GRAMPY"

Jesus called you to bring you home,
Up to heaven where the angels roam.
Although our tears could not make you stay,
You are with us still, everyday.

Paradise is what you left to find,
Grief is only for those left behind.
A whole year has past, but our tears still fall,
We wonder why God had to call.

Life was much happier when you were here,
We would give anything to have you near.
But you are in heaven where you belong,
Listening to the angels hum Jesus a song.

Even in death love does survive,
And our love will always keep you alive.
I know the only sadness you feel, is not
Being able to end our grief, but never look back,
Because we have belief.

Belief that we will all be reunited again,
Belief that there is no more suffering where there had been.
So we will wait here and fight the tears that we cry,
Because it is we will see you later, never goodbye.

Know that love is a bond that death cannot sever,
We love you and miss you today and forever.

GRAMPY,

Two years have gone by could it really be true?
Two years have gone by sadly missing you.
The world seems dim without you here,
Although your gone, we sense your near.
Watching from Heaven with so much love in your heart,
Even death cannot keep us apart.
To see you again would be like a dream come true,
Not a day goes by that we are not with you.
We do not know how, we do not know when,
But we are one year closer to seeing you again.
Life seems so gray, time seems still,
We wanted you forever but it wasn't God's will.
So here we are to tell you once more,
How much your loved, you know it, I am sure.
We were not ready to let you go on ahead,
There were still things that needed to be said.
Like how without you the sky has gone gray,
And how there is an emptiness everyday,
And at night your on our minds, you fill our dreams,
There is a void in our hearts, that gets bigger it seems.
The world holds no solace, no comfort, no hope,
It seems so grim, so hard to cope.
Because our family has been separated, only a temporary split,
but there is a missing piece of our puzzle, and only you have the piece that fits.
Time has no comfort as days pass on by, your time was up and only God knows why.
Never wanted to give you up, we never had the choice,
You had to move ahead when Jesus spoke his voice.
He called your name you could not hesitate,

You looked back once but you could not wait.
You were greeted in His warm embrace, He wiped your tears right off your face.
He brought you comfort said we would be okay,
That you could look upon us everyday.
So you went ahead although we had to part,
You left behind your mark and a piece of your heart.
We each carry it with us it's always there,
There were so many things you were able to share.
So do not worry, do not regret,
There are so many things we could never forget.
So there are only a few things left to say,
The ones we tell you everyday.
It is only right to love you,
It is only right to cry,
It is only right to hold you in our hearts and to never say goodbye.

SADLY MISSED TODAY AND ALWAYS,
BY CHRISTINA CHICKLOWSKI STAPLES

This poem was written for my sister on her wedding day. My sister has always taken care of me. She is by far one of the most special people in my life. I could never ask for a better sister. She was married when I was eighteen and it was very hard on me when she left. But I wanted to tell her how much she meant to me and how much I love her so that is why I wrote this particular poem for her wedding day.

In my beginning you were already there, changing my diapers and fixing my hair.

It was you Joey and I, the trio of three, we were built in best friends, the way it should be.

We played our childhood games, that made memories to last, it feels just like yesterday, could it really be the past?

You knew so much like mom number two, Dad and Mom called you mother hen, and the name suited you.

As being the oldest you played your role, helping us and guiding, and taking control.

I looked up to you and the grown up things you did, it was like you knew everything and I was just a little kid.

When I cried you held me, when I was sick you cared, everything you had you gave me, and we shared.

We all grew older and we still stayed close, but the built in trio seemed to be becoming a ghost.

I watched your make-up and your teenager shows, I was a tag along with your friends, and I was stealing your clothes.

Time kept moving and we find ourselves here, I feel so much inside I could burst into tears.

I am so happy for you and all you'll receive, I never thought you would actually leave.

Our family of five, now expanded to six, were gaining and losing, what an odd mix.

I hope all you have is happiness and health, and I couldn't have chosen a better husband than if I chose him myself.

I'll miss walking down the hall and into your room, without you the house will hold some gloom.

I'll miss Christmas mornings, when I jump on your bed, I'll miss when I can't sleep how you'd pet my head.

I'll miss making you and mom laugh in her room at night, not having you with us just doesn't seem right.

The house will seem empty your presence will be missed, and there is so much more to put on this list.
But as we grow older things have to change, even if it hurts, or seems really strange.
This is your time, and you have to go, happiness is all I want for you, I just want you to know.
It's hard to believe your leaving home, it's hard to put eighteen years inside of this poem.
I anticipated this moment for so long, and now that it's here I have to be strong.
What you have is true love, now take it and go, I love you much more than you'll ever know.
This is where your new life will start, happiness for you is flooding my heart.
You have so much ahead so follow your dreams, reach for the stars, or whichever one gleams.
Go now happy knowing you're blessed, know in your heart you deserve the best.
You gave us all what you could give, my only sister go now and live.
Tricia, my entire life you were at my side, I love you my sister, the beautiful bride.

This poem was written in honor of my wedding day. It was the happiest day of my life.

It was one of the easiest poems to write and my favorite.

My favorite because when I read it I can remember a time when I was happy. When I am feeling down I like to look back on that time and try to remember that there are times when I do feel good.

*Today is the day we start our new life,
Joined together as husband and wife,
We started off young everything new,
And together in love our relationship grew.
An attraction that blossomed into romance,
I am only glad we took that chance,
We have been through laughter, we have been through tears,
We started off as kids dating but matured through the years.
We have grown together through each year,
We have grown so close that we find ourselves here.
Today is the day we wrote it in stone,
We will walk through life together instead of alone.
A bond so close, a connection so rare,
A oneness, a unity that we share.
Once we were halves together were whole,
Were linked in mind, heart, body, and soul.
The love we have so true, so deep,
That when one of us feels pain, the other will weep.
So many journeys, so many tests,
But together we made it through all of the quests.
In our hearts our love is strong,
A connection so close we could never be wrong.
Feelings of joy so sincere,
Together now we have nothing to fear.
I have found my soul mate now my heart has wings,
You never know what joy life brings.
I have my partner, it was meant that we'd meet,
And now I feel that my life is complete.
So blessed is our day by the heavens above,
We are bound together by eternal love.
Thank you for joining us as our journey starts,
Know you are always close in our hearts.
When life gives us rain we bring each other the sun,
Once we were two, but today we are one.*

This poem was written in honor of one of my best friends Kelley Dasso Devantier for her wedding day. Kelley, Kristina, and I have been best friends for twenty years and I wanted to tell her what she means to me. They say if you can count the number of true friends on one hand than you are lucky. So than I am extremely lucky. So Kelley here is to twenty years of laughs, tears, and an amazing friendship.

DEAR KELLEY,

Where do I start? there is so much to say, I can't believe that it is your wedding day.
It seems just like yesterday that Barbie was the bride, and that we never left each others side.
Sleepovers every weekend watching movies Kristina didn't like, rollerblading and riding bikes.
Kick ball games, and soft ball too, I did not do basketball I still need to make that up to you.
The memories are endless, so many laughs! Whether it was making up dances, or the Hampden Beach rafts.
We started off little girls and formed a lasting bond, with dreams of flying fairies, mermaids, and magic wands.
It started out so simple, we based are friendship on dolls we shared, and through the next twenty years on how we cared.
No one could understand our thousand laughs or private jokes, like the Spanish toy we do not know who broke.
We helped each other through the bad times, we had our share of fights, but mostly wonderful memories of laughing through the nights.
Every weekend was a new adventure, the chipmunks sure had one! I have so many heartfelt memories that I could never pick my favorite one
We have our trips of camping when Kenney would eat sand, but I remember turning to each other when no one else could understand.
Every first experience a crush, a dance, a kiss, we stuck it out together those youthful days I miss
But I remember mostly that we leaned on each other when times were rough, we stuck together through childhood, and all the teenage stuff.

We stayed close when we were trying to stand on our own, and even though things changed we were never really alone.
Growing up you were my second family your house felt like it was mine, and growing up we hit rough patches, but our bond stood through time.
It seems like that was just yesterday that we were little girls, laughing at our likeness with dresses dolls and curls.
Well these three little girls, are all grown up now, and fate has kept them together somehow.
But time has moved on and here we are today, to honor you and Chris on your wedding day.
I am so happy that you met him and how things turned out, life is funny how it twists and turns, and how fate comes about.
I must admit that it was hard to let you move away, but I knew he was good for you so there was nothing I could say.
It still seems strange when I call you that your not down the street, but God had these plans for you and Chris to meet.
We are sisters by choice, friends by chance, but this is not an excuse to do our spice girls dance!
Know that even though your states away, and were miles apart, our friendship will always be number one within my heart.
There are so many memories people could never comprehend, it would take my whole life to write them down although your worth it my friend.
I am so happy to be here and celebrate you becoming a wife, I wish you and Chris a loving and fulfilling life.
Just know when days go by and we cannot find the time to talk, you are still in my thoughts and prayers, and every step I walk.
I am so happy for you both, I hope all of your dreams come true, and Kelley please know my life was better just from knowing you.
Congratulations ! I love you with all of my heart!
—Benny

This poem is based on a painful experience in high school. A painful challenge, losing friends that you love.

In high school you believe the friends you have will always be there and that it will never change.

But you cannot prevent change, people grow up. They want different things, they change.

And they are not always willing to give you that extra mile. They are not equipped with empathy to stand next to you, but I don't blame them. Such is life.

When I look back on this poem I can still remember the pain, I thought everything around me was crumbling. I survived. It was hard because I knew I was different from everyone.

But this time I knew being different made me a better person.

Not everyone sees things the way I do, not everyone feels things the way I do.

This was just another lesson on being "special."

You don't talk to me like you used to do,
You don't help me with what I am going through.
You used to tell me your secrets and call me on the phone,
And now you pulled away from me leaving me alone.
We walked down the halls together laughing as we'd go,
Now you either walk right by me or wave a passing hello.
What makes you think your better? When I was their when you wept,
You no longer want to know me, I am someone you no longer accept.
When one of us had a problem, it became both yours and mine,
And we'd work it out together until everything was fine.
I fixed your problems when you were sad,
I did everything for you, I gave you all I had.
Now I ask myself why you won't help me in return?
I guess that was a lesson that I had to learn.
I was the one you came to when you were excited or glad,
I was the one to calm you down when something made you mad.
Now my heart is feeling heavy, that our bond has been erased,
And just because I am sick, I had to be replaced.
It proves that you are shallow, only concerned with you,
All you care about is being liked, and becoming cool.
Your family was like mine, your house was like my own,
And now that is someone else's second home.
You really use people to get what you want,
I guess I did not know you, you manipulate and taunt.
Now I listen to you as you brag and boast,
And because I am different, to you I am a ghost.
And it's not fair, that I am a phase or spurt,
You act like it doesn't matter,
Even though you know it hurt.
Now your new best friend comes before me on your list,

And sometimes I feel like to you I don't exist.
And now my heart has a big empty space,
And it's so sad knowing someone else took my place.
At the time it seemed that our closeness would never end,
But because I am sick I am no longer your best friend.

Some people just journal their thoughts I do the same but in the form of poetry. I write poetry to cope with the day to day changes in my moods. You will see it for yourself. The different periods of which sometimes change so rapidly it's like hitting a brick wall at a hundred miles an hour. It comes out of nowhere and hits you so fast that you never saw it coming. That's what my day to day life is like. Never knowing if it's going to be a life threatening crash or just a day on cruise control.

It sucks, but it is what it is. I just sometimes wish it was a crash test dummy in the car and not me. But no man can choose his destiny. And this is my destiny and all I can do is shake off each accident that sets me back and climb back behind the wheel and face this illness head on.

And that is just what I am doing one mile at a time.

In almost every poem I speak of putting on "my show."
My show to me is a brave face. Acting as if nothing is wrong as I do most of the time. I can't tell you the countless days at work, with friends, family, parties, everywhere, that I act as though I feel fine.

I rarely do. That is why I speak of it so much because it can be draining hiding your real feelings.

To me it's almost easier than explaining the real ones.

The real ones are so different from everyone else's in my life. So just to let you know that "my show" makes me stronger because to you it appears that there is nothing going on, I consider it a compliment that I am now able to function so much better that I can keep my feelings under control to act out "my show."

I hate how in life things have to change,
I hate because it hurts, it is abnormal and strange.
Your loved ones die and your left behind,
Locked in a depression, searching for peace in your mind.
I remember the good times they seem so far away,
You would give anything to go back to that day.
And tell them the words that you regret you didn't say,
You didn't say them because you didn't know they couldn't stay.
Memories are good that is all that can last, with comforting
Times that are left in the past.
You wish you could once again be a child,
With no worries but school, so simple so mild.
But before you know it time marches on,
You missed out on some dreams, and those years are gone.
There were so many things that you wanted to do,
But your illness got the best of you.
The illness came full force with attack,
And those days of your youth you can never get back.
There were so many things I thought would be accomplished by now,
But getting through everyday life is an achievement somehow.
This was not what I dreamed, what I had planned,
But I no longer drown in anger, I am just learning how to understand.
I do not feel sorry although some do not believe,
I cannot change this, it will not leave.
I do not know why people think you have control,
The brain is just as complex as the soul.
When someone gets psychically ill, do you tell them to stop it? Like they have the free will.
I do not search for sympathy, just acceptance I guess,
It has taken me years to learn to express.
Fear held me back, afraid that they would judge,
And I am trying hard to let go of grudge.

It is not their fault, some just are blind,
They believe you have control of the mind.
You do to a point, but they do not see,
That your thoughts have you trapped and you cannot break free.
You have trouble telling if what you think is real,
Are you just being paranoid? Tell me what to feel.
I manifest things in my head, hard to admit
I believe them true, and do not like it one bit.
Because how can you tell if it is real or fake?
You trust no one, is that a mistake?
You think everyone is talking about you,
You do not want to go outside,
Admitting you are not normal will diminish your pride.
One minute your laughing, the next your enraged
Not sure what has happened, why it had changed.
Some days just running errands is like the whole worlds weight,
You feel just exhausted, you cannot see straight.
You cannot sleep without meds, your thoughts keep you awake
But then the next morning you feel the meds are a mistake.
You could sleep the whole day,
You keep gaining weight, it just makes you more sad,
Then you get resentful, insecure, so mad.
How is it supposed to help making your self image bad.
Then you see models skinny on T.V., then you just wonder
Why can't that be me?
You can hardly function to work, so money is tight,
So much more stress, it just doesn't seem right.
Then you see people you know,
They think you are fine, because you put on your show.
Their are days I feel good, but I know they won' last,
For a little while, but comes back full blast.
Your used to it so you just trudge on through,

You're a trooper what else can you do?
You want to give up so many days,
But the bad ones do pass, although the illness stays.
But the good ones are worth hanging on,
I know it is hard but you have to be strong.
Because you are here for a purpose, what I don't know.
Maybe to save a life? Have children? See them grow?
Life is a gift just hang in to find out,
Learn how to live, what life is about.
You only get one chance do not throw it away,
Survive off of hope and you will get through each day.
And when the burden gets heavy, and you feel all hope is lost,
Just one more day to laugh is worth what it cost.

In this poem entitled "MY FINAL FAREWELL" I was preparing to die.

I was giving up, I planned my death and was working up the guts to do it.

As you can see I never did. All because of a promise I made to my mother.

And also because I thought back to all the laughs and smiles I endured in my life.

All the moments I enjoyed, and although at this time all I felt was pain, I made it through.

And yes it came back numerous times, but it also left again. I laughed again, I enjoyed things again. Had I followed through I never would have felt those feelings again, and those feelings were good. Don't get me wrong when the feelings are bad, they are rock bottom fall into darkness bad. They are I feel as though I am never going to get up again or feel good again. But I did. And yes it always comes back and haunts me all over again with the same tormenting spell, but it always leaves for a little while and gives me that brief break that allows me to enjoy life again. And during that time I love life. That is what I try to remember and hold onto during those dark times in which the disease is so relentless with it's scorn. But when it eased up I created memories that I wouldn't have that my family wouldn't have. I did not want to share this poem but my feeling is, if I can show you that I made it through my darkest hours, maybe it can give you the courage to do the same.

This is my final farewell,
My hurting is just too great,
Although you may have tried to help me,
You were just too late.
I don't know why I had this illness,
I was so misunderstood,
I needed you to help me,
But you never could.
You could not save me from myself,
Although I wished you could,
I am sorry that I let you down,
But I warned you that I would.
I know that this was selfish,
But I could not take more,
I wish I had the answers,
I wish they had a cure.
God gave me this so I think he will forgive,
It was just becoming way to hard to live.
I felt so alone, although I knew you were there,
But you could not stop it, although the burden you did share.
I just wanted to apologize to my mom and dad,
You were the best parents I could have had.
And I am sorry mama, I couldn't take this pain,
It would roll in like the thunder, and down pour like the rain.
You knew it all to well and I am sorry for all the grief,
I tried so hard to be positive and carry that belief.
Belief that it would get better, belief and lots of hope,
But this illness stole my life from me and I just couldn't cope.
And I am sorry teddy you were the love of my life,
I wanted things so different, but I could not ease this strife.
I want you to remember me but please stay strong,
I want you to have a happy life and for you to move on.

You were my everything, I loved you more than you could know, you gave so much happiness, although it did not show.
The days we spent together made my days complete,
And when one day God calls upon you, once again we'll meet.
I never wanted to leave you, but I could not survive,
It was such a struggle just to be alive.
I don't really know what's out there but it must be better than this, although I will long for you in heaven, I will always miss.
Tricia and Joey take care of mom and dad,
I know it will be hard on them, tell them I am sorry that there sad.
I love you both so much I am sorry if your mad,
You were my closest friends, you often made me glad.
Glad for all the memories, even when we'd fight,
Please just remember me, and pray for me at night.
I was so lucky to have you, you made my world a better place, hopefully God will still love me, forgive me with his grace.
Tricia how you'd comfort me, and Joey how we'd laugh,
I did not stand a chance though, you can do the math.
And I know that it will be hard, I took away the third,
But think of me with angels, flying as high as a bird. And I did not want to throw it all away,
But I hurt so bad every day.
Mom and dad, I do not know what to say,
Except that I am sorry that it turned out this way.
I will long for your comfort, for every hug and kiss,
And although I hope to be with God, your who I will miss.
No one was like you, your comfort was what got me by,
I just longed to no longer feel, to no longer cry.
Although I will cry for you until we meet once more,
I will await the day I can hold you again, although when I am unsure.
The love in my heart was so great, but God gave me this burden, the illness played my fate.

I too will long for you, that's the pain I will still have to carry, but the illness needed to die, that I had to bury.
I know I promised to never do this, it's not really what I wanted, but how the bipolar mind manipulated and taunted.
I wanted to live, but the illness took that from me,
I had to get away from it, I had to be set free.
To Kelley and Kristina, oh what good friends,
Although we have parted our friendship has no end.
I know you will be angry, I know that it will be hard,
But this was the hand I was dealt, and I did not have a winning card.
I wish I could have reached out to you, but it was much to hard to explain, sometimes we have to walk alone, and endure a lonesome pain.
I just wanted to thank you both for all the laughs and smiles, please just remember me, think of me once and awhile.
And know I will still be with you, although I will be gone, I will look upon you daily, I am sorry, I was wrong.
And daddy I will miss your storys and all our heart to hearts, although I won't be in this world, we will never be apart.
You were the worlds greatest dad and I am thankful for the bond that we had.
All the comfort you gave me helped me to last a little longer, but I did not have it in me, I thought that I was stronger.
I want you and mom to forgive me, I am so sorry for the grief, I tried to stay positive, but there was no relief.
Perhaps for a little while, but it always came back,
With a vengeance stronger every time, for all the days it lacked.
The love in my heart was so great, I just hope you can forgive,
And I will try my hardest to give you the strength to live.
Please do not feel anger, regret, or guilt,
There was nothing more you could have done,
It's the way my brain was built.
Just pray I get to heaven, because I felt this world was hell, I love you so much, and I am sorry,
But this is my final farewell.

Forgive me for what I want to do,
Forgive me please for being blue.
I try so hard to put it behind,
But you do not understand, it haunts my mind.

And it is there for life it is there to stay,
I do not want it here, but it will not go away.
You call me crazy but you do not see,
How it eats away at me.

But I understand I am too much stress,
Too much to handle like all of the rest.
My disease is different, too powerful to be real,
It affects my life and how I feel.

It is invisible to the ignorant eye,
They think I can prevent this suffering cry.
I want to be normal, I want it so bad,
I am so alone and so desperate,
And so heart wrenching sad.

They think I can change it, but I have no control,
It has been there since birth, inside of my soul.
When God created me he added in this,
With a sprinkle of love, and a heart warming kiss.

This pain has driven everyone away,
And there is no one strong enough to stay.
It is not there fault, I know in my heart,
What will not stay hidden, will drive us apart.

*I am a good person this I know, if this is what I have
Been given, I must accept it and go.
I feel so helpless, so alone inside,
And nothing will ease it, not even the million tears I have cried.*

I feel alone, I feel sad,
Everything in my life seems to be going bad.
I am drifting farther from all I know,
I tend to hide, I try to let it go.
But I am growing weak, falling weary,
I can't seem to see things clearly.
Falling into darkness all over again,
I am so used to this place, it's where I have been.
Been since the start of my days, it doesn't leave,
No matter who prays.
Comes back with it's vengeance, relentless, no relief,
I can't stand it every month! It torments me, brings me grief.
So time keeps passing, and I want it to end,
There is no way to connect, not a soul,
Not a friend.
I feel such a burden, it's heavy, hard to carry,
I want it to suffer, die, and to bury.
No one to reach for, no one around,
I want to escape to heaven, but I am earth bound.
It's tormenting, awful, and mean,
You could only know if you have seen.
Seen it through the eyes of the mentally ill,
Who never had a chance, who doesn't have the will.
The will to keep fighting this losing battle,
I am adrift in the ocean without a paddle.
I want to know happy, know it once more,
I want to get out, but I can't find the door.
So I weep alone, in a pain so bad,
No human on earth should have to feel this sad.

*I know I think slow, my reactions are slow. I can see it I know you can.
I don't know how to fix it I don't have a plan.
I know it's this poison I put in my body,
The poison that gets me through when I am confused and spotty.
I can't concentrate, my thoughts fly away, I can't pay attention,
I do not make sense with what I say.
I say stupid things that make me cringe, I have remorse in my heart with
a guilt ridden twinge.
I am so overwhelmed. I struggle through the weeks,
No one hears the sputters I speak.
I can't really express I can't put it in tongue,
I no longer feel happiness, I no longer know fun.
My life seems wasted, I don't have anything to do,
What a waste of life, and dreams that fail to come true.
So much depth in my thoughts that no one sees,
Such lonesome feelings, such ignored pleas.
Such lonesome times, Such misunderstood tears,
Such judgement calls, and unwanted jeers.
What gives you the right? Who do you think you are?
Do you think you are better? That you will get far?
I know the world better, I know it so good,
You think you do but you never could.
You do not see it through distorted eyes,
I see it better, without all the lies.
I see the pain, I see the truth,
Although from sensitivity,
I was denied my youth.
I felt things different,
I saw the true colors,
I felt the pain of all the others.
I cried more than I laughed,
I didn't see the glass half full,*

I had a massive burden to pull.
I felt you looked at me funny,
I thought I was strange,
I had to fight my thoughts,
They had no range.
They would take me to far off places,
Make me afraid,
Show me scenarios,
As I prayed.
I thought they were real,
Maybe some were,
To this day sometimes I still am not sure.
I sift it out like noodles that you strain,
All because of a defected brain.
If I did not take pills I would stay up for days,
With idea after idea, and thinking up ways.
Ways to make up for my unhappiness,
Forgetting how much I am blessed.
I hate myself, although I try to not,
There was much I wanted to do,
I wanted to see a lot.
But bipolar held me back,
But I guess that's okay,
I can't change it now,
There is no way.
So I will end here,
No longer complain,
About this disorder,
That haunts me in my brain.

Here we go again, right back on the same spot,
I don't know what's the matter but I am hurting a whole lot.
My soul is sadly aching I have such a heavy heart, and no matter how hard I am fighting it the tears and sadness start.
I try so hard to hide it. I feel so out of place, but look deep into my eyes and you'll see it on my face.
The pain I am feeling now is nothing that's brand new, but when? I always ask myself will it finally be through?
Each day gets harder and harder, and I struggle to win this fight, I sit here and wonder if I will ever be alright.
The suffering is unbearable, I feel it when I sleep, the pain is so intensified, it's endless wrenching and deep.
I see how life is precious, but I don't want to be alive, I want it all to end yet I struggle to survive.
I see my dreams unraveling, my life is fading fast, and I feel like I have nothing but heartache in my past.
I know there is so much good in life, I want this hurt to drop, I want my life so different but I don't know how to make it stop.
I saw all of my plans diminish leaving me with none, and why when I had so many, the illness could not leave me one?
It's taking over my life and filling it with ache, and why when I have so much good does my life feel like a mistake?
I've let my life slip I feel foolish and dumb, but my hurting is too great, I hate who I've become.
Why my life is like this is so totally unfair, and why when I know they do, does it feel like they don't care?
I feel my time is being wasted, in life you get one chance, why is mine being wasted in a depression's trance?
No one knows about me, I hide so they can't see, someday can't I be happy the way I am supposed to be?
If it takes forever I'll still be waiting then, please somebody save me I am hurting again…

In some of my poems of depression things were so severe that when I look back I almost scare myself. I still get like that at times, but when you are feeling better and you look back it is scary.

The emotions were so intense it could have been very easy to give up. But I have been doing better so it was worth hanging on to get to this point. I get through the depressive episodes by hanging on to advice given to me by someone very special. It's very simple.

"It will pass and you will feel good again." and although at some point or another it always comes back, I know it will leave even if it is for a short period of time.

And although this day on which I am writing this has been a hard one, I have had severe paranoia and delusions and anxiety today I am living it out. That is all I can do. I so badly want to sleep to escape it but my racing thoughts will not allow it.

So I have been struggling through today and I am getting through it on the hope that tomorrow may be a better day.

So all of you out there that is the best coping mechanism I can offer, I hope maybe it might work for you, I can only hope these words may change some of your own self destructive thoughts.

I can only hope for my friends out there, I hope that just might be enough.

SOMEBODY TELL ME WHY?

YOU KNOW SOMETHING IS WRONG WHEN IT HURTS TO SMILE.
I WONDER IF THE PAIN WILL STOP? EVEN FOR JUST A LITTLE WHILE.
A SECRET THAT YOU TRY TO HIDE, BUT THE PAIN IS SO INTENSIFIED.
I WONDER NOW WHY I AM HERE? TO FEEL ALONE? TO SHED A TEAR?
WHAT IS GOING ON INSIDE MY HEAD? WHEN I CUT MY WRISTS IT IS TEARS I HAVE BLED.
I WANT IT GONE, I WANT CONTROL,
IT DOES NOT UNDERSTAND IT IS MY LIFE IT STOLE
NO MATTER WHAT I DO OR SAY, IT IS THEIR FOR LIFE,
IT IS THEIR TO STAY.
MY HEART IS SO HEAVY MY EMOTIONS TOO STRONG,
WHEN WILL I ESCAPE THIS HELL? I CAN'T HANG ON TOO LONG.
I TAKE MY PILLS, I DO WHAT THEY SAY,
BUT NOTHING CAN STOP ME FROM FEELING THIS WAY.
I GO TO BED CRYING I WAKE UP DRAINED,
I GO ON SUFFERING FEELING TOO PAINED.
BECAUSE OF MY BEHAVIOR I DRIVE EVERYONE AWAY,
I CANNOT CONTROL IT BUT I AM THE ONE TO PAY.
I SILENTLY SUFFER FOR AS LONG AS I CAN,
THEN THEY LEAVE AND I AM ALONE AGAIN.
YOU CAN'T PUT IT IN WORDS WHAT GOES ON IN YOUR HEAD,

THEN YOU SCARE EVERYONE WITH THE WORDS THAT YOU HAVE SAID.
IT HURTS TO GET UP IT ACHES TO LIVE,
WHY IS THIS SOMETHING THAT HE WOULD GIVE?
WHY AM I CONDEMNED TO PAIN?
WHY INSTEAD OF SUNSHINE DO I SEE RAIN?
IS MY LIFE'S PURPOSE TO SUFFER AND BE SAD?
I WANT TO KNOW WHY I HURT SO BAD.
WHY WHEN I AM IN PAIN DO PEOPLE HURT ME MORE?
THEY USE AND ABUSE AND KICK ME TO THE FLOOR.
HOW COME NOTHING EVER GOES RIGHT FOR ME?
WHY WHEN I LOVE SO MUCH DO THOSE PEOPLE SET ME FREE?
I GAVE ALL I HAD I GAVE ALL I COULD,
THEY CALL ME CRAZY BUT I AM MISUNDERSTOOD.
WHY WHEN I START TO CARE DO THEY THROW ME BEHIND?
IT KILLS MY HEART AND WOUNDS MY MIND.
I BLAME MYSELF MY SELF HATRED KILLS,
I SEE THE BAD THINGS IN MYSELF, AND THE PAIN JUST FILLS.
I DO NOT UNDERSTAND WHY NO ONE REALLY LOVES ME WHEN I LOVE THEM SO MUCH,
SOME ONE TELL ME HOW TO STOP THE PAIN,
WITH AN INTENSITY THAT THEY CAN'T TOUCH.
WHY AM I MEANT TO SUFFER? WHY CAN'T SOMETHING FOR JUST ONCE GO RIGHT?
IT'S LIKE I AM IN THE DARKNESS, WHEN EVERYONE IS IN THE LIGHT.
NO ONE COULD UNDERSTAND ANYTHING I FEEL,
AND IT MAKES ME SO FRUSTURATED THAT ALL OF THIS IS REAL.

WHEN THERE IS SO MUCH GOOD IN LIFE, WHY DO I FEEL SO DOWN?
WHY DOES IT HURT TO SMILE? AND FEEL SO NATURAL TO FROWN?
SOMEONE TELL ME WHY THIS IS THE LIFE I HAVE BEEN GIVEN,
I DID NOT GET TO CHOOSE,
NO MATTER HOW I FIGHT TO WIN I CONTINUE TO LOSE.
I AM TRYING TO ACCEPT THAT I AM MEANT TO BE ALONE,
I WANT TO CONTINUE TO TRY, BUT I HAVE TO GO ON MY OWN.
IT MAKES ME SO MAD THAT I CAN'T GET AWAY,
AND PLEASE TELL ME WHY I ALWAYS FEEL THIS WAY?
I AM FRUSTURATED AND I AM ACHING,
NO ONE CAN HEAL MY HEART, SO IT GOES ON BREAKING.
I SILENTLY SUFFER, EVERYDAY I CRY,
I GUESS IT'S MEANT TO BE THIS WAY, BUT CAN'T SOMEBODY TELL ME WHY?

All alone I will stand and wait,
Until peace arrives with the hand of fate.
The tear drops fall one by one,
I have no where to turn, I have nowhere to run.
Lost in despair, lost inside of gloom,
Inside I feel hopeless, inside I feel doom.
With no one's hand to reach and take,
For I fear they to will be fake.
So I sit alone and wonder why?
Why is it that I hurt and cry?
Will my turn arrive with joy?
Or will this pain continue to toy?
Toy at my bleeding heart,
Until the tears and rages start.
Then abandon me alone and weak,
With no sane words left to speak.
Stole my hopes, and stole my smiles,
Put a few more records on my files.
Left me confused, left me to hurt,
Left me with death again to flirt.
So much anger, so much rage,
Acted out on my life's stage.
It came out of nowhere, out of the sky!
And I just want to know why? Why me?
Why this despair? This mental pain is just not fair.
Terrorizing, haunting, agonizing pain,
Too much for any person to contain.
They get mad and they start to yell,
But I am the one in this mental hell!
Trying to be normal, trying to win,
Trying so desperately to fit in.
They think I am weak, but I am who is strong,

I just do not think I will ever belong.
It is something no one wants to see,
That is hiding deep inside of me.
This is my destiny, so I must continue to fight,
And keep praying that one day I will be alright.

SOMEONE

Please tell me someone why I am hurting so
And make this hurting stop,
Please someone calm these tears,
Calm each and every drop.
Please someone tell me why I am so unhappy when todays a brand new day?
Please someone stop these heartaches before they waste my life away.
Please someone tell me why I feel so all alone,
Please someone explain all of these feelings, before their forced to be shown.
Please someone stand by me in my hour of need,
Please someone take me by the hand, please explain these feelings,
And please someone understand.
Please tell me when this happened, why did it start?
Why is my soul so sadly bleeding? Why do I have such a heavy heart?
Please stop these painful heartaches, too unknown to be heard,
When inside I am screaming but I am too silent to form a word.
Please someone help me, it's just too much to bear,
Please someone notice, and please someone care.
Please someone get me through this, it's just too much to take,
Please someone hold my heart together because it's starting to break.
Please someone tell me why I feel so worthless, please tell me why I am so hard to love, Please tell me why I am someone that no one is thinking of.
Please someone take away my rain and give me the sun,
Please help me someone......................

I awake in the morning and get ready to go,
I throw on my smile to put on my show.
My heart is bleeding my soul is sad,
I start with doing favors,
So I can ignore this pain that hurts so bad.
I think about others, I listen when their upset,
I concentrate on their needs although mine are never met.
Ignoring the held back tears piercing at my eyes,
I keep on smiling, filling my head with lies.
No one seems to notice, no one seems to care,
And while I am cheering them up, it really seems unfair.
I silently suffer what else can I do?
I can't think about me I have to think about you.
If I think about me I feel the depths of despair,
That's just too hard to cope,
I feel lost inside loneliness with no glimmer of hope.
So I keep on going showing a brave face,
I've become so good I don't seem out of place.
But when I am alone and I start to think,
It's like a ship in the water that's starting to sink.
I feel so outraged, I feel so much pain,
The loneliest tears fall fast just like rain.
So finally still suffering I go home and I cry,
And all I ask myself is the question why?
Why is it their with no purpose but pain?
Why with all I have am I being sucked down this drain?
So intense are my feelings of anger and hurt,
So intense is my sorrow when I see the wrist of my shirt.
Scarred and bloody with my feelings and more,
Will I ever feel better? My heart isn't sure.
In my life's journey depression has always followed along,
This earthly life is just somewhere that I'll never belong.

Sad today not sure why, I feel empty and alone inside.
I feel so lifeless it's hard to move, tired I guess trying to get back in the groove.
Today is my first day back after a week, but my spirit is falling to be listless and bleak.
I am so overtired it doesn't seem right I can no longer sleep soundly through the night.
Tired of anxiety, tired of fear, sick of this paranoia that makes my thoughts unclear.
Why won't it ever end? I wish peace was something that man could send.
But here I am lifeless and weary, in a world that feels so dreary.
I don't want to fight I am in a bind, I feel like I am going out of my mind.
How can one escape their self? It seems unlikely with this deteriorating mental health.
I am fighting so hard I am struggling through, but who can I tell? Only you.
Only these pages on which I express, the depths of my thoughts on my loneliness.
I don't even want to see my husband or any one at all, but I can't get around that, I can't make that call.
So sick of questions that have no answer, you can't see this like it's diabetes or like it's cancer.
It's their in my brain not a soul can tell, it's working it's hardest to keep me in hell.
I need to stop thinking about every component, that keeps me from living in the moment.
I don't always have to work on getting well, it's hard enough to keep it in this shell.
A shell where the dark secrets hide, that are no longer being denied.

My feelings are no longer protected, no more worries of feeling rejected.
I know myself and that's all I need, you can figure it out yourself with these pages that you read.
God gave me a trial, but gifted me in return, he wants me to reach out to others, and help the ones that yearn.
Yearn for acceptance, so they won't feel alone,
The gift of understanding, that feels too unknown.
So when they read these pages they will know too,
That I am somewhere out their with them feeling how they do.

My vision now is so much clearer,
If you could look through my eyes and see the distorted mirror.
I realize now that I am on my own,
Locked in my thoughts, forever alone.
Trapped inside this negative hell,
Desperate to be happy and well.
Having no one to tell, having no where to turn,
Desperate for someone to understand and learn.
I cannot make them it is all free will,
Won't anyone care about the tears that consistently spill?
Everyone is just out for fun,
But believe I am the one who wants to run,
Run far, run free, run as far away from me.
But I am stuck for life, there is no escape,
And my heart has been beaten, and is out of shape.
Tired and dragging, hurting and worn,
Scarred and forsaken, hopeless and torn.
No matter what I cannot seem to hide,
The tracks of the tears that I have cried.
The anger inside continues to build,
That this is my life and it is not free willed.
There are so many days I want to give up and die,
But I know that I can't so I just scream and cry.
Each day is a struggle, life seems like a curse,
No one wants to be around me and that hurts even worse.
Each day I hurt someone new that I love,
Will the pain ever stop? Or only in heaven above?
I will wait for my day when peace will arrive,
Then I can truly enjoy being alive.
I sit here in anger, I sit here in rage,
While I am writing the tears are dripping onto the page.

The tears are so lonely, so misunderstood,
I want to be happy, I know that I should.
It is so unfair, no one knows,
This is not the life I would have chose.
My internal hell is breaking my heart,
My mind has been driving me crazy since my life's start.
I want someone to help me but I do not want it known,
Please someone help me, I am so alone.

I wish you could fully understand what I had to endure to grow,
I wish you could feel the depths of my heartache so you could know,
Then you could know what I went through, this path I took,
It was not filled with butterflies or a bubbling brook,
More like volcanoes of rage and bumpy unpaved road,
With no direction or compass with a three hundred pound load.
No one to walk with, to lead or guide, no one to share my fears or with whom to confide.
With fear of not understanding what was going on,
With so many people who were there and then gone.
So much confusion trying to find direction,
So much neglect, so much rejection.
I didn't know how my brain would react next,
I didn't understand why and I felt so perplexed.
Their was no one there who shared my thoughts,
Who could understand my sorrow, or call the shots.
It was so confusing I was so misjudged,
And of my youth I was begrudged.
It was always lonely I didn't understand,
I was lost in the desert, a resolute land.
I went to doctors I took my pills,
But I was deprived of youthful thrills.
Instead they were filled with tears and sadness,
Then the next moment with rage and madness.
It happened so fast like the flip of a switch,
Almost like a computer that has a glitch.
One second I was me the next someone I did not want to know,
I did not want the world to see but I could not help but show.
Then I would be abandoned for what I had no control,
I did not ask for a damned soul.
It was given to me I did not have the free will,
I begged for it to be taken back, but it is with me still.

I was chosen to bear this cross, although because of it I have endured great loss.
But it also has given me open eyes, to feel empathy when one cries.
I have so much emotion in which I am learning to contain,
I have grown use to sorrow and pain.
My thoughts take me places I don't want to be,
They show me visions I do not wish to see.
I can't express it, because you are different from me,
People reject what they cannot see.
They think that your just sad, no big deal,
But they have no clue how you think and feel.
They say to get over it but there is dysfunction in my brain,
They really do not know what I fight to contain.
Can I help it that it doesn't work right?
Can I help that I am tired of this fight?
They judge for what they are not educated about,
If it were up to me I would have chosen a different rout.
Because ignorance is so well known,
I overlook it although I feel alone.
Because if you were educated maybe you would see,
That there is really something not right with me.
I just wish someone would care to learn,
Then maybe someone would show some concern.
Because it is so lonely this life that I lead,
Understanding is something that I still need.
So please do not pass judgement on what you don't get,
I am tired of feeling angry, and having regret.
So unless you are educated do not look at me and think you know,
Who I am and what I have endured to grow.

Bipolar Disorder what's your purpose?
Why torture me? Why the ruckus?
Why do you deliberately alter my thoughts?
Oh how you deceive with your tormenting plots.
Why do you cause me to see different from everyone,
We could look at the same thing but I am the only one.
To see it distorted, to not here it the same, your who I
Hate, you're who I blame.
Instead of reassurance you give me fear,
You make me second guess, and why is unclear.
You cause me to fight its real, no it's not,
I never understood but you never taught.
You left me to question, paranoid as learned,
That you are in my brain,
You are etched and burned.
I sometimes feel like I am not in my body, I am not really real,
I see visions of things and I believe what I feel.
Then I can't tell when they really are,
You cause me to run, but I never get far.
You can't run away from the depths of your mind,
The visions you show me, I cannot go blind.
The things I hear, I cannot go deaf,
There is no escape, because I cannot choose death.
So tell me what I am supposed to do?
It doesn't work very well co-existing with you.
I try to fight you but your strength is great,
I feel like I have too much on my plate.
Why do you want to continuously disrupt my world?
Why do you feel the need?
I think I have suffered enough,
How much more must I bleed?

Will you ever let up?
My pills help me fight,
You torture me in the day,
And even worse at night.
Why do you twist my thoughts and give me rage?
I have no exit for my feelings,
No compensation no wage.
There is no outlet no one to tell,
I feel you are laughing,
When I am not doing well.
I cry all the time,
My emotions overflow,
But you won't explain why this is so.
Why did you choose me?
I deserve an explanation,
I am on a path with no destination.
So I guess I will fight you off,
Just continue to try?
I just wish in my heart you would tell me why.

Sick of life,
I want to know death,
I would feel such relief to draw my last breath.
And to not know this world any longer,
I don't feel well,
I don't feel any stronger.
Only lonely only scared,
I have nothing to do,
I am so not prepared.
Same old thing a different day,
I know longer feel the strength to pray.
My life to difficult, as I am tortured within,
I know in my soul that I cannot win.
I have no outlet, no way for it to be known,
I am in a time machine, a different zone.
I feel so depressed and I don't know what to do,
I wish a cure was something I knew.
But I don't have the answers, I don't have the heart,
I wish I did but I am not smart.
All I do is try to cope,
And it's frustrating,
As I sit here and mope.
I don't feel like I am coping,
The depression is thriving,
I just keep on pushing,
I keep surviving.
But I don't have it in me to keep on going,
I have no one to call,
The mania is showing.
I can't believe the act I put on,
I seem so normal, I seem like I am strong.
When really inside, I don't know who I am,

My thoughts fly away,
They burst through a damn.
They surround me, drown me while I fight,
I struggle to swim,
This just can't be right.
They fly away like balloons,
That I struggle to catch,
Bring them back to earth,
They scatter as I fetch.
They will float away so I hold on tight,
I hold on with all of my might.
Sometimes it seems easier to just set them free,
What's the use not a soul can save me.

Why is your brain demented?
Why is it that your tormented?
Where did it come from?
Who would have sent it?
I hate that my brain makes me hate being alive.
I hate that for a "normal" life I have to strive.
I hate my thoughts, how they race and flow
They torture me why I don't know.
I sit everyday struggling through,
But I can't sit and tell all of you.
Because you could never comprehend a day in my shoes, it's more than just a case of the blues.
I sit here and analyze, every component,
Every shape and size.
I don't know I just hate my brain,
I hate my feelings and all they contain.
Because everything hurts me, I think so weird,
I can't seem to function, I believe what I feared.
I can't trust you, paranoia has control,
I know you will hurt me, I know in my soul.
Rage has subsided, but obsessive thoughts,
It could be about anything, how my brain rots.
It's rotting inside it remains unexpressed,
You would look down upon me when I am giving my best.
You could only comprehend if you were on this road too, searching for direction, when you don't have a clue.
All I know is that I am tired I want to let go,
This brain is something I don't want to know.
Don't want to walk on this path, this lonely road,
I am lost and confused, it's too heavy of a load.
This can't be my life, why this mind?
I wish that I could hit rewind.

And find the time in which it went wrong,
And I would fix it, and still be strong.
I never had a chance, never had a choice,
Couldn't speak my opinion, couldn't speak my voice.
If I could have I would have begged to be free,
Free of this illness that is killing me.
When one looks upon you they never know,
What lingers inside what you don't want to show.
I appear to be normal but I suffer so bad,
I wish you could know my pain and the struggles I've had.
Then you would know me, really know who's inside,
Then maybe you could sit with me through this roller coaster ride.
Trying to balance is so hard between depression and anxiety, it has no disregard.
It doesn't care how you suffer, doesn't care how you feel,
I just can't believe this is my life, please don't let it be real.
I want to live my life to the fullest, always a hit never a miss,
I want to live my life in sheer bliss.
But that's not what I was given what else can I do?
Just sit here and wish that I was normal like you.

I feel depressed again,
I am feeling useless,
Without a friend.
What else is new?
No one to tell,
I am getting agitated,
I am starting to yell.
I feel so sick,
I feel so blue,
But I play it off so well,
That no one has a clue.
I am tired that this book is all I have,
To express myself as things get bad.
Sick of this illness, it never stops!
It calms for awhile, then the hurricane drops.
It comes through and destructs my whole world,
Then it blows over leaving everything mangled and twirled.
It comes in just as fast as it leaves,
Destroys everything in its path and it's so hard to believe.
It comes with no warning, doesn't make a sound,
Then it throws everything off, and shatters steady ground.
Just when you thought storm season was gone,
It just comes barreling along.
Cuts off your provisions, cuts off your air,
Leaves you in chaos, with nothing to prepare.
Your dreams have been shattered once more,
That you could be normal, but you can't close that door.
You can barricade it, but it has no lock,
No key, no storm door, it destructs with shock.
It's useless, it can only be contained for so long,
Then it comes back and it is just so wrong.
What do you know?

Paranoid again,
Don't trust you,
Don't trust where I've been.
Fuck you brain!
Tired of your shit,
And all you contain.
Tired of dragging,
Tired of trying,
Tired of lagging.
Sick of hiding the tracks of my tears,
Sick of these thoughts, manifestations and fears.
Funny you see, they do not no me at all,
Don't want to help me up when I fall.
Tired of this poem, tired of you,
Tired of this life and feeling so blue.

I have dreamed about escaping,
I am dreaming of a gun,
To escape this forsaken world, wouldn't that be fun?
To pull the trigger and feel my brain splatter,
It would not be tormenting me, this illness would not matter.
Then my soul would leave behind this sadness,
No one understands me, not an ounce of gladness.
No one cares to know me, they tell me to pretend,
I do it all the time, for the sake of you my friend.
I want it all to end, I just want to die,
So I don't have to sit here, lonely as I cry.
Embarrassed of who I am because you belittle me,
No one cares to listen no one cares to see.
I can't hide who I am but you expect me to,
I struggle to hold it in, you don't know what I go through.
But why would you care? So continue to ignore,
It is not your life, not your journey to explore.
You don't want to walk with me and I can't expect you to, I wouldn't wish
it on an enemy, it's just something I go through.
Lonely and self absorbed is what depression is,
It's a daily test, and sometimes a pop quiz.
Pop quiz number one, can you survive the day?
Pop quiz number two, can you conceal your feelings away?
Can you sit there and act like you feel fine?
For the sake of others while you are tortured in your mind?
Sure you can, so what else is knew?
You do it so well that no one has a clue.
You appear normal just what you aimed for,
No one knows a thing about what you endure.
You can't give them a glimpse into your world,
You are a rare kind, they will poke and prod you,
And judge before they find.

They don't want to know you, they just are not the same, it's hard to love what's different, I can't give the blame.
Just like I am different, they don't have the skill,
To want to know, to want to help, it is all free will.
Maybe they do care, but that's the way there made,
To turn there back, to walk away, maybe that's why they never stayed.
You make a statement they don't comprehend the meaning, although for some understanding the proper word is pheening.
Yeah I long for it, but acceptance has won,
But I still dream of escaping,
I still dream about a gun.

I do not want to feel,
I wish that it was gone,
How much longer must this hurt go on?
I hurt myself on the outside, because I hurt within,
But I will not let it defeat me,
I cannot let it win.
Things have been so hard,
The pain, it hurts so bad,
I long for some normalcy,
I long to not be sad.
The paranoia is so hard,
But at least I recognize,
But still I long for someone who can sympathize.
I think about the past, I have so much guilt,
And the fact I cannot change it makes my heart wilt.
I am begging for some help,
I am longing to escape,
But how do I know it's real?
I sense that you are fake.
But they tell me different,
That it's all inside my head,
Oh how my heart has suffered,
Oh how my heart has bled.
How I long to die so I don't have to feel,
It seems so inviting, but I can't make it real.
Because I am in pain, it seems to be my ticket out,
But I don't know what death is, or what it's all about.
I would rather be a part of this world, although I am in pain,
Because you just get one chance,
Although mine feels insane.
There is so much that I want to do,
Although the illness takes that too.
I guess things could be worse,

Although I can't always see how,
So I will continue with my act,
And at the end I will take my bow.
And know that it did not conquer me,
Although it broke me down,
I got up again, I won it all around.
If I can win each battle,
I just might defeat the war,
Although each day is a struggle,
And I can't take much more.
But all week long, I thought about death,
Such a peaceful journey,
But not my job to accept.
It's not my choice, I must wait for fate,
Although the prospect can seem so great.
But I keep going, I break through,
I prove I am strong and you can too.
So each day is a struggle we know that too well,
We are trapped inside a horrible spell.
But each day we get through,
Is like acing a test,
Keep up your strength, your giving your best.
So here I am to tell you once more,
Keep on fighting although the battle wounds are sore.
So whatever your quest, whatever your story,
Keep on going, we will have the glory.
The knowledge of something, they could never know,
We are just special, with a burden to tow.
So just keep on living, just give it a try,
Because although you don't want to feel,
You don't want to die.
So pick yourself up again, although you feel unsure,
You haven't lost a battle, so you have won the war.

There is no comfort, there are no smiles,
I am not getting anywhere and I have been walking for miles.
On this lonesome road with ditches,
I fall and get up, it's smooth and then switches.
I am alone I can't even talk,
This life is such a lonesome walk.
I walk alone and beg for a friend,
I am in a maze that does not end.
A friend who goes through what I do,
A friend that knows this maze to.
A friend to pick me up when I stumble,
Who doesn't criticize or utter a mumble.
Who wants to help me as I weep,
A friend who knows what I keep.
Getting through life is such a struggle,
As the acting gets better as I hide and smuggle.
I smuggle my real feelings that drag me down,
I put on a smile right over my frown.
I am so paranoid and no one understands,
I don't want to either, as I sit here and plan.
Plan for a life I am not destined to live,
No matter how much I give.
I am meant to suffer it is what it is,
It was not my choice it was his.
It must have a purpose, although I can't tell,
Why would he condemn me to hell?
I know I say that all the time,
But I don't see happiness or the sunshine.
I only see a life destined for sadness,
Although sometimes there is gladness.
There are good times, some good days,

But when that is over oh how it pays.
Pays me for what I missed,
It laughs at me and I get so pissed.
It makes up for everyday it was gone,
It is sometimes absent but for never to long.
It's funny you see,
I hide it and no one knows me.
The only way they could tell the only way it would show, is
if they read these pages then they will know.
That my life is no picnic,
It's an involuntary ride,
With no one to sit with or whom to confide.
Each day that I get through is like a reward,
Although the pain is a piercing sword.
Killing me little by little,
While I try to balance in the middle.
Keep on acting as though you are fine,
Hide those tears stay in line.
No one hears, cares, or knows,
But that is my life and the way it goes.
So keep on going, keep on running,
Although the pain is often stunning.
Know your good, know your strong,
Just keep on going although the roads long.
You'll get through it you always do,
And maybe one day it will ease up on you.
So hold up your head, keep walking tall,
And know that you will get through it all.

As usual I feel abnormal,
Like a key that doesn't fit,
As usual I feel alone,
And no one understands a bit.
Don't tell me your like me because your not,
Because you do not hear, like your out of earshot.
Do you know what it's like to have no one to understand?
No one to lean on? Or to reach for their hand?
I cannot express my thoughts I cannot confide,
You act like you care about what lingers inside.
Have you ever been educated on the mentally ill?
Would you ever take the time to learn about a pill?
If you stepped into my shoes you would know my pain, but you only think of yourself, doesn't that drain?
I have never met anyone so selfish in my days on earth,
Have you ever thought about others since the time of your birth?
If you're my friend than you should have known,
What brings me pain, what makes me feel more alone.
But you sat there and did not speak a word,
My useless speech must have never been heard.
You only call me for advice, you never think of my heartache, never think twice.
I knew I had no one, and it makes me more sad,
Not one true friend on earth to be had.
I guess I just feel betrayed, because part of me thought you listened, but I was played.
Silly me I should have known, I always felt different as I have grown.
I don't connect with anyone really,
Not at my level,
I am a loner, I am a rebel.
I am rebelling against those who use my heart,
Who only care for themselves,

As it tears me apart.
I could call you up but I hold back,
What's the use understanding is what you lack.
Not enough compassion to walk in my shoes,
I would think you could have solved it I left enough clues.
There are so many signs, I wish you cared enough to see, that there is an endangered species, and the species is me.

The tears keep on falling to the floor,
Always wanting something more.
From these feelings and thoughts I want to flee,
Won't my mind ever let me be?
Send me to the wild, send me to the abyss,
Just so I don't have to feel like this.
I will never be okay I am tortured deep inside,
Something that I am no longer able to hide.
Negative thoughts flood through my brain,
Always causing unwanted pain.
Tears fall as frequently as one will blink,
Why does one have to think?
How do I get these thoughts to end?
Happiness is something I can not pretend.
Torturous thoughts continue to flow,
How can I get them to go?
Suffering all day long in my head,
I long to be free, I long to be dead.
Once your dead the thoughts are gone,
No more wondering how to go on.
Always sad in my head all alone,
Wishing for a positive tone.
These tears I am to tired too cry,
Tired of wondering how I will get by.
I want to give up, I don't want to try,
How can I feel this way? I want to know why!
I do not know why this is so,
Peace is something I long to know.
I feel so foolish thinking happiness could be ours,
Everytime I look at my scars.
Scars of anger scars of rage,
Brought on by my mental cage.

When my mind is blank I will feel I have won,
But for now I want run.
The tears continue to drop,
I just don't know how to make it stop.
I can no longer put on this show,
Please God, just let me go.

Paranoia is one of the hardest things to endure in this illness. Sometimes I feel like people are thinking bad things about me, or there talking about me, then someone will tell me there not that it's in my mind and I just have to accept that and try to talk myself out of it. It rarely works. Thoughts pop into my head and I will think everyone is mad at me. I think up scenarios and obsess about it so much that I think it's going to happen or it has already happened.

Then I start to trust no one, like there all out to get me.

Then I get anxiety from obsessing about things that happened years ago that I cannot change. I don't know what to do besides cry and keep it to myself because I know it's not normal.

I know people see glimpses of it and since they do not understand they think I am weird and probably pass judgement.

I am learning not to care what they think. They could never understand and I can't expect them to. Their brains do not function in the same manner. But it just makes this illness more challenging, difficult, and as I always say very lonely. I wish I knew someone that I was close to that could relate and not think I am weird.

I can't help it, I just have to live with it. It is very challenging and draining. But it is just another part of this illness that I must endure and learn to conquer so it does not conquer me.

And that is what I am doing one day at a time.

In these poems of rage some were brought on by comments made by people I love, and jut to see how one comment can be analyzed and affect my whole train of thoughts and feelings can be very depressing. One little thing can lead to a downward spiral, that's when my sensitivity because a problem. Some days I have rage just because. I hate the rage mostly because I do not feel like I have control of myself or the emotions.

It just builds until it explodes and there is so much behind it that it feels uncontrollable. In the poems of rage the wide variety of what causes it, what I express is an example.

It's everything, I become a walking time bomb and I never know when or where it will come out. Sometimes I act absolutely crazy in front of people that I would rather not have a glimpse into my problems. But it just goes to show the lack of control I have when the rage attack comes on. In my rage episodes is usually when I hurt my loved ones the most. I say horrible things, some things I will not remember. I can only hope they can find it in there hearts to forgive me and know that is the illness that takes over, and that it is not me, and that I am sorry to cause them pain, just because I am in pain. But I never realize until after the rage is gone. Then I cry guilty tears. So thank you to my loved ones who still go on loving me regardless.

I hate it that this is the way it is, the way it has to be, but there is nothing I can do but deal with it the best way I can, and that is what I am doing.

I thought I saw them following me around,
But when I looked back all I saw was the ground.
I thought you could read into the depths of my mind,
So I tried to clear it, to see what you would find.
I thought you were angry I had to have done something I am sure,
I thought I heard a knock on my door.
I see scenarios playing, I can feel the pain,
Then I convince myself that it's not real,
And I start to feel insane.
Why is my mind so different from yours?
Why does it open to different realms, dimensions, and doors?
Why won't it stop when I feel so sick?
Why does it always have to trick?
I don't like it, I would like to stay footed to earth,
And not fly away with the questions of life, death, and birth.
Why is it my thoughts fly away?
They scatter keep rising, can't catch them today.
Why is there this heaviness inside again?
I realize what a fool I've been.
Did I really think it was gone for good?
I wanted to believe although I didn't think I should.
I am so agitated, so alone,
I need someone to talk to,
Someone who's known.
Known my heartaches, known my pain,
There isn't a soul out there, oh what a shame.
How sad, how lonesome to never connect,
I guess it's pride, and the will to protect.
I don't think that you'll get it, that you'll ever understand,
This complicated soul that I am.
So I sit here lonely as my thoughts scatter,
With no one who can help me,

Because it's not like I matter.
The only thing that matters is that you are doing fine,
Why would you care that I am out of my mind?
So I will just sit here with these visions that I have seen,
And wish that I was normal, at least I can dream.

Another day I sit in a rage, my only way to cope is to write on this page.

I hate that they cannot understand, I hate it more that they don't try,

I guess they are not considerate I guess that they just lie.

I am one in a million but it hurts inside, everyone is so selfish, and to understand I have tried.

How are you all such jerks? Why don't you care? With your greed and smirks?

Am I the only person alive that feels different and scared? How are you so two faced? I guess I am not prepared. I thought growing up that you thought like me, but I was wrong that is plain to see.

Although my brain is dysfunctional, I am almost in better shape, because to be so self centered is a

Disgusting mistake. Because when you need me I refuse to be there, only considerate when you want me to care. I don't want to sit here and revolve around you, I am not just here for you I am here for me too. I don't want to help you I want someone to help me, I am not your psychiatrist and I don't work for free.

If you had it your way I would be at your beck and call, well guess what I do not want to help you at all.

Because when I ask I get the cold shoulder, and my heart is angry resentful and colder.

Don't want to sit around and please all of you, I am surprised this is something that none of you knew.

Oh how cute you thought you should come first, when you would not spare a drop of water to satisfy my thirst. Guess what I am done! Sorry to have ruined all of your fun! Guess what your pathetic and weak,

Too selfish to reciprocate to listen when I speak.

And no I am not just a spoiled brat, it is so disgusting listening to that.

It just proves that I am not heard, not even a single word.
I am not surprised it is expected you see, why would you give a damn about someone like me?
I guess I have a different idea of a friend, I do not sit here and just play pretend.
And hope that you will pity me, I don't want your pity, I no longer care if you see.
Because in my heart I know their is a reason, I accept it more with each year, and each new season.
I know you don't want to sit their and hear me out, in my fits of rage, tears and shouts.
Because you are not capable to want to learn, I accept it although I still yearn.
But to sit there and hear what you really feel, I know you are a manipulator, my trust you want to steal.
Because you want it to benefit your greed, somehow it ends up getting you what you need.
You sit their and judge but you never step back, to see your faults, and the compassion you lack.
I guess its easy to point the finger, but you do not know my pain and how it will linger.
But do not make comments about things you barely know, it makes you look ignorant, as you act out your own show.
When I yell at my mother it is not about her, it is between her and I why your involved I am not sure.
My mother stands by me no matter what I do, yes that's unconditional love, something you probably never knew.
She lets me yell when the emotions overflow, something you do not see, so you could never know.
I am her child she sees me in pain, she lets me get it out when it can no longer restrain.
I know what it must look like to others, that I am bratty, abusive to my mother.

But she knows the truth, and I know too, so I don't know why it is a concern to you.

Because she is all I can count on when I cannot bear, she loves me protects me, she is always there.

Obviously my mother knows I am mentally ill, I have enough guilt for a lifetime that cannot be cured with a pill.

So do not sit their and criticize, and act like you love me with your judgement and lies.

I do not care what you think I do not care what you say, you act like this is a game that I want to play.

Because you have no idea what goes on behind closed doors, you don't know the anguish, you only think about yours.

Do not accuse when you don't know the truth, I have had these problems since the start of my youth.

Guess what its genetic I did not make the call, I did not ask for it, its not for attention at all.

I do not use it to get my way, I cannot change no matter what you say.

Dou you think I want to be plagued by torturous thoughts? You do not know how I feel I can't call the shots.

Is it a crime to be loved or even spoiled? you do not know my suffering or how I have toiled.

So do not go around and act like you love her, because you are so ignorant to judge a book by its cover.

I am a bird that should not be caged,
I cannot fake it, it cannot be staged.
Why lock me up and throw away the key?
Why hurt and torture me?
You do not know me nor do you try,
You do not care too, and I don't know why.
It hurts it aches as you keep me away,
Locked in this cage where forever I stay.
My mind is caged, so why my soul,
Is to belittle me your lifelong goal?
Manipulate that's what you all do,
You don't care to know what I go through.
To you people I am all in the wrong,
Keep it up and I will be gone.
I will not support you I will be absent like you,
Don't know the meaning of a friend that is true.
So get out, out of my sight, because the way you view me isn't right.
You have me pegged all wrong, tired of hurting and struggling along.
You're a tool, a fucking joke, never heard a word I spoke.
You don't need me? See if I care! Time for reality you better prepare!
I will be gone in a second, a flash, thanks for ripping open another gash!
Why would you care that I bleed? As long as you have all that you need.
Guess what? All I'll leave behind is dust, I will be out so fast like wind with a gust.
See what you'll do then,
I look where I am going not where I've been.
See you hope it was great! I am through I am straight.
All I hear is how evil I am,
You rub salt in my wounds and don't give a damn.
So fuck you, you let me fall down,
You left me to drift, you left me to drown.
Don't want to hear you, your fake fucking words.

Don't feed it to me go feed the birds.
You will get what you want from them,
They won't have an opinion on getting screwed again.
They will sit there, they don't have a voice,
Just what you wish of me, but it isn't your choice.
Only want to hear me when I am happy and smile,
You want to bail on me at the sight of tears,
Kinieving and vile.
Then you burden me with words of abuse,
Not because you love me, because you choose.
Try to twist my feelings and my mind,
You think I am stupid but I am not fucking blind.
So put me down if it makes you feel fine,
You can have the glory, go ahead and shine.
I will sit here I am not right,
I cause every heartache, each nasty fight.
That's what you want me to believe,
Oh you are sneakey, how you deceive.
I see right through you, I am not dumb,
Although to your ridicule I am now numb.
So sit their I will have the last laugh,
It's fifty fifty you do the math.
Don't want to listen don't care to hear,
I am rock solid just to make it clear.
So keep throwing knives, you are missing my heart,
You cannot aim for shit, try to restart.
So thanks again I love you too,
I hope you know the anguish you put me through.
So see you later, don't give a damn,
It's just sad to realize you don't know who I am.

Always about you, disgusting so gross,
I now know why I can't get close.
I don't trust any of you and I never will,
You bring me so much hate and regret that I can't sit still.
Always about what you want and need, filled with so much self absorbtion and greed.
And now that I defend myself I am a bitch.
But your greed and betrayal caused that switch.
And I couldn't be happier standing my ground, not letting you use me like a dish rag that you just throw around.
Because I am a person with feelings that you should not abuse, I am not here for you to walk all over because you choose.
I have so much anger that I can't let go,
You did such a number on me and you do not even know.
But I am glad that I am stronger because if you screw me again, you will get a taste of reality and what should have been.
So do not sit there and act like your words don't drain
You have no right to say them after you caused me so much pain.
I could sing like a canary after all that you have done,
You don't even remember not even one.
But if I could go back you would get it times three,
Then you would know what you have done to me.
So don't act like your better than everyone I have known,
Because if I had been smarter I would have left you alone.
And where I wonder would you be? Certainly not a friend to me.
So thanks for the deception I hope it was fun,
Your dumb ass thinks that you have won.
But I know so much more than you think,

You should be the one paying my shrink.
Your so sickening that you still would never see,
All the pain and agony.
Hope it was worth it you will pay your whole life,
It's great to get stabbed in the back with a knife.
Not just once but over and over again.
Oh that's right it never happened, spare me the deception
That it's all in my head.
See how you twist it and you lie,
You never cared about my heart and how you made me cry.
It must be nice to be you and never sacrifice,
But I will make sure that you pay the price.
Because my heart is so wounded, it's not even whole,
You stripped me of my dignity and broke down my soul.
So much anger I cannot let go, because honesty is something that you do not know.
Because I think of how much I gave,
You think it's a free pass I will just let it wave.
Don't think you have me fooled I can see straight through,
I was just kind never a fool.
You all think your so smart that you have me in your web tightly spun, but I am to quick I am not dumb.
In my world trust, there is no such thing,
I see how you try to gain it what you are trying to bring.
Bring me in a world where you can break me down,
But you're all so stupid you look like a clown.
Because I know what's up I can detect, my heart is something that I will protect.
You all make me sick you are evil and should be locked in a cage, just another day and a case of rage.

Wouldn't it feel great to not worry? Wouldn't it feel great to not cry? Wouldn't it feel great to sink into a black hole and die?
I don't want to feel these tears pricking at my eyes, I don't want to answer all the why's.
I feel like I am drowning in a dark abyss, so sick of the tone and listening to this.
You don't care about me just keep packing on my stress, keep giving me more so it leaves you less.
I am drowning deeper in this place, I am putting up a wall, just to fill the space.
It's so lonely here, dark and filled with doom, there is no such thing as sunshine, or a twinkle from the moon.
You never seem to care, so I wish I didn't anymore, I wish I could feel my blood dripping to the floor.
And feel the life slowly drift away, their would no longer be sorrow or a reason for the pain to stay.
And then I could finally know that peace does exist, I don't feel it here it's something that I missed.
Keep pushing my buttons, keep putting me through stress,
You will be the sorry one for loving me any less.
Keep hurting me with your words it will not get you far, I will just add it to each and every scar.
Scars caused by your selfishness, it's always been about you,
It's so sickening I can hardly believe it to be true.
So sit their smug thinking about yourself, because in heaven I will have wealth.
Wealth of love and compassion, and not an ounce of pain,
I will no longer flirt with death, the illness will no longer drain.
So just sit their and continue to use, it's not worth to fight, argue, or accuse.
So I will let you absorb inside yourself, so what else is new? You could care less about my health.
It's not my place to judge you will be for your sin,
You cannot break me down, so you will never win.

I sit here and wait for the tears to spill,
I sit here dieing, in pain still.
I am so tired, so stressed out,
so depressed, not sure what about.

A dark cloud follows me around,
Fatigued and useless, my head just pounds.
Disconnected from everyone, I want to be happy,
I want to have fun.

This burden I carry, too heavy of a load,
I just sit here and wish for my brain to explode.
No more thoughts to drive me insane,
No more wandering down depressions lane.

I want to die, so I do not have to feel,
Everything seems fake, I do not know what is real.
Where is my smile? Where did it go?
I feel so empty, but who would know?

How much longer do I have to stay on this road?
I feel like my life is on repeat mode.
I do not feel like a person, only physically ill,
But I do not want to take another pill!

I know that they help, but I am dieing inside,
They say life is a gift, but oh how they lied!
I am in internal hell, there is no one to help,
There is no one to tell.

Heaven is a place no sorrow no woe,
That is the place where I need to go.

A peaceful eternal sleep, with no thoughts to think,
And no sorrow to keep.

Peace throughout eternity, heaven is the place I long to be.
I have suffered now it needs to end,
I no longer want to play pretend.
Because even when I am happy it waits for when,
It can return full force and crush me again.
I am sitting here writing, but I feel I am not here,
I am in a different realm, which one is not clear.

I need help, but I am to exhausted to try,
So I will continue to sit here longing to die.
I wish I had a gun, so I could kill my thoughts,
It would feel so good to fire those shots.

And lay there and feel this despair slip away,
And be happy not to wake up sad everyday.
I guess I am supposed to suffer, cannot take the easy way out,
No one even knows me what I am about.

But I will sit here and not speak a word,
Because even if I tried to explain I would never be heard.
I know I am different, I am on my own, I will just sit in my world,
All alone.

I wish an angel could swoop down from heaven,
and take away this pain. And show me the sunshine,
And leave behind my rain.

But that dream is never coming true, I must endure this suffering,
What else can I do?

I cannot sleep anymore and it angers me,
My thoughts keep me awake,
Making me crazy you see.
The rage has subsided,
But anxiety in its place,
What's the use,
I show a brave face.
But I like to sleep it gives me a break,
Gives me a rest from the pain I must take.
I take a little every day,
Some days more than others,
Some days seem so gray, some with vibrant colors.
But I need my sleep to escape my brain,
Because if I don't get the break I start to go insane.
I am tired you see but my mind is going,
The thoughts are racing, the anxiety towing.
It's making me nuts although it's not showing.
I am getting so angry, I am getting so pissed,
I have no one to express it to and it's a lonely twist.
Lonely and angry and almost neglected,
No one understands it so it's rejected.
I want to scream it out,
But no one would care so I silently pout.
And get so angry that I want to break everything in sight,
Then maybe someone would help me and know I am not right.
But why would you care when your life is fine?
Your brain functions, you don't have delusions in your mind.
I am not blaming you, just angry at your lack of care,
I would for you so it seems so unfair.
So I just go on being ignored,

Going out of my mind, consumed so bored.
I am bored of this illness, won't it ever end?
It's like a consuming draining unwanted friend.
Thanks for this illness although it was fate,
Being tortured daily just feels so great.
I would trade anyone for some mental health,
So bipolar disorder go fuck yourself!

Is their anyone out there who knows me at all?
Is their anyone that feels my tears when they fall?
Is their anyone out there who is not too selfish to know,
That I am not well although I can put on a show.
Thanks for the compliment that I function so well,
Thanks for not hearing that I go through hell.
Why would you hear? When Your so absorbed in you?
You might think that you know me but you do not have a clue.
Don't pretend like you care, because you really don't,
I don't care if you notice because I know that you won't.
I am so sick of listening about all of your woe,
Your self pity is sickening and you do not even know.
So concerned with yourself that you cannot even see,
That I am a person living with agony.
And no not everyone feels the same,
If you actually listened you would know you are lame.
I don't care if you know me, and you do not either,
So I have decided to take a breather.
Because guess what? My life doesn't revolve around yours,
And caring for you is not one of my chores.
I am so sick of being sucked dry, tired of listening to your petty cry.
Grow a backbone and get out, don't call me up and cry and shout.
Don't tell me words that are not cared to be heard,
Because from now on I do not say a word.
Because it is all about me, see how you like me then,
Don't sit there and act like you know me my friend.
All you know is that you can cry on my shoulder,
But my sensitivity for you is growing colder.
I do not need you I get by on my own,
Its all about you as you have shown.
So we are disconnected a weaker bond,
But the next time you need me I will not respond.

Because I will be tending to me, your selfishness would be great to see.
Sitting their getting so pissed because you won't come first on my list.
Your so self absorbed you don't have a prayer,
It must be nice to be too selfish to care.

Do you know what it is like to be lonely?
Do you know what it is like To not know who's real and who's phony?
Do you know what it's like to feel like an unknown breed?
The only one who really feels emotions, and cares what YOU need?
I live in a bubble I am not like you, I feel things intensely I do not think how you do.
I can walk in your shoes and feel what you feel, but I cannot determine what is fake and what is real.
No one cares like I care, no one feels my pain, no one understands me what I contain.
I am a different species that is unknown, one that is so different it does not care to be shown.
Sensitivity seems like a curse, not a worthy trait, empathy also has sealed my fate.
It hurts me that they don't understand but I guess that's the price, you can hurt me once but never twice.
I get so paranoid I make up scenarios in my head I still believe they are true from comments that are said
But how do I know that they are real? I determine this through how I feel.
Am I strange or is everyone fake? I feel that opening up is a severe mistake.
Weakness is enjoyed that's how they thrive, they do not care how you struggle to survive.
Because you don't really know them, and they don't know you, yeah it is lonely, but what can you do?
Open your heart to people and get stabbed in the back? Because they will do it and that is a fact.
There are really repercussions when you betray my trust, I hate deceit, greed, and lust.
I am not perfect, but I don't find it hard, to be a person of honor, when you let down your guard.
I sit here and think what we will go through in life, I can't handle loved ones dieing, suffering, or their strife.

We will all grow old and watch everyone die, why do I want to hang around and cry?
I cry enough in my bleeding mind, searching blindly for strength to find.
But I guess I am strong because if you thought like me you would also suffer in this eternity.
In feelings that are to intense to understand, would you cry at the grocery store for a fellow man?
Would you feel guilty for looking at someone, because their was a chance that you made them uncomfortable by your sidelong glance?
Do you cry for the handicap because others laugh? This behavior is not normal you do the math.
But that is what is wrong they do not care enough, they are not capable to handle this stuff.
So I guess that makes me special, but I feel alone and sad, I carry life's sorrows and the burden is bad.
It seems that I pity myself, but it is just hard to bear this mental health.
After awhile it weighs down your soul, but I guess it is worth it to pay heavens toll. Suffering on earth is rewarded by God, he will carry me to heaven, while I leave my heart ache beneath the sod.
And it will feel so worth what it cost, although on earth my soul feels lost.
I do enjoy earth I love so much, my family, my husband, a loving touch.
I love more clearly than people know how, it is just tiering to accept it now.
It is so hard to accept that people can be true, I hate lies and deception but that's thanks to you.
Because you say one thing and do another, is that how you treat a fellow sister or brother?
Fill your head with lies if it helps you sleep at night, because I can see right through you, I see the true light.
I love more than your whole existence could contain, I can stand with you and feel your pain.
But most do not have the empathy to give me that back, obviously empathy is what you all lack.

And it took me a while to understand, not everyone is programmed to extend their hand.

Selfishness takes over that is plain to see, but is their anyone out their at all like me?

Look away as the tear drop spills,
Or as I slash my wrist,
Or as I swallow a bottle of pills.
You read me all wrong, you don't even know,
What's inside my heart, what I try to show.
You don't even know me, you never try,
And every time you judge me I want to die.
I want to die so this pain disappears,
I want to die, to run away from my fears.
Fears that this is it it's not getting better,
I want this earthly life to severe.
Then the pain will be gone, it couldn't survive,
Not if I was no longer alive.
But it's not fair, don't want to give up my chance,
My dreams, my wishes, my journey, my dance.
But it follows me every where I go,
And it's hard, not letting it show.
I want to scream it! I am sick of hiding!
I want to get off this roller coaster I am riding.
All by myself up and then down,
Screaming all alone, no one around.
The highs and the lows, the dips and the dives,
So gruesome and extreme, and how it thrives.
Thrives off my fear, thrives off my racing heart,
It won't let me get off, didn't tell me when it start.
So all by myself around and around I cry,
So can't you understand why I want to die?

Do you know what it's like to have a depressed heart?
Unsure where it came from, and when it did start?
I feel so lifeless, so lethargic and out of sync,
There is something missing, in my brain, a link.
A link that provides normalcy and controls emotion,
Instead my feelings cascade like the ocean.
Angry and wild and uncontrolled crashing,
Sometimes calm, sometimes lashing.
So dark, so blue, an unknown deep,
With many secrets to hide, too many secrets to keep.
The world sometimes finds comfort in it's depths,
While I sometimes struggle to take breaths.
It grabs at me, so icy cold, and tries to pull me down,
With a death gripping hold.
The current so strong drags me out to sea,
I feel like I am drowning,
And no one can see.
My mind is like the ocean unpredictable and vast,
A storm can brew out of nowhere and destruct your path.
Its energy is strong it takes over with ease,
Then the next moment it's as gentle as the breeze.
But oh when it's angry you can feel its scorn,
It sucks you in its loneliness, it can leave you so torn.
You don't know day to day, you can never predict,
Will it be calm like the bay? Or will it leave you adrift?
You cling to your life raft, no provisions, no strength, no direction, no hope, too much length.
So dreary when it begins to rain, leaving you in such unwanted pain.
Throwing you crushing you as you drown in the unknown,
This ocean so heart breaking, in these depths all alone.

Here I am another day, searching for comfort,
Trying to find my way.
I feel so lost, so un amused,
I feel despair, so confused.
I want life, everything it has to offer,
It only gets harder, I wish for softer.
I am not destined for greatness, only to suffer,
I guess it's supposed to make me tougher.
But I feel so lost that's the only word,
But I feel like I go on unheard.
I appear like I am just like you,
When in the depth of my soul that is untrue.
I hurt, I ache, and pretending is my own mistake.
All the things I want to do,
I will never conquer my dreams with no thanks to you.
I am fat because of you, I am destitute, I am blue.
I can't see the world because I don't have the means,
I can't follow through on any of my dreams!
I don't have it in me to go to the store!
I feel like my life is one giant bore.
Everything costs money, I can hardly function to work,
And because of my paranoia, I act like a jerk.
No one understands me, I feel alone and scared,
I was thrown into this and I wasn't prepared!
I feel sick all the time due to these pills,
They help fight you off,
But deprive me off skills.
Skills that I need to function in the world,
Then if there touched I am tossed and I am hurled.
People look at me strange when they catch a glimpse,
But I know in my heart that they are just wimps.
They couldn't take a day in my brain,

One moment and they would be laying there slain.
But not me, I live it, I tame you well,
Although I admit it has been hell.
The manifestations are great,
The delusions are fun,
The paranoia gives me the incentive to run.
The agitation makes everyone yell at me and get mad,
The rage was the best, everyone left me when things got to bad.
The depressions wonderful, no will to live,
What a kind present to give.
You really shouldn't be so generous,
No you're really too kind,
Thanks to you I sound like I am out of my mind.
But I am more real, I am more aware,
And all the judgment is really unfair.
But bipolar it's just as you wish,
I will not live in bliss.
Sure I will have good days in between,
But that's where your kinieving and mean.
But I will battle you until death,
I will still be battling when I take my last breath.
So let's keep going with these battles and duels,
I don't have a choice, you make the rules.
You were the one who invaded my brain,
Didn't ask my permission, but in society I take the blame
So I will keep going that's all I can do,
And hopefully one day I will overcome you.

I guess it would be easy to give up,
I know it's easy to self destruct.
But yet I keep moving,
I keep going,
Not sure where this path leads,
Where I am going.
I know I feel like I am not in my body,
Like I am not here,
Is everyone like that?
I know what I fear.
My fear is that I am different,
I know it all to well,
I hide it, you can't see it,
I do not tell.
I can't explain it, because the look in your eyes,
You look afraid, like I am full of lies.
Maybe your afraid, that you could be like me,
Maybe your afraid of the reflection you might see.
I am outside myself, how do I get back?
Before it comes full force, with it's vengeful attack.
Do you know what it's like to have your thoughts fly away?
Scared of what you think? Afraid of what you say?
Do you know what it's like your moods up and down?
Constantly, daily, no steady ground.
I am not like everyone but that is okay, my mind plays tricks,
Everyday.
I sink into dark depths and have trouble coming back,
The next moment I could be normal, the next I sink into the black.
I see things distorted, but now I realize, like a hall of mirrors,
It's difficult to recognize.

But acceptance is important, acceptance is key,
Although it took me quite awhile to see.
I don't want this, I never did,
I always knew it was there, even when I was a kid.
I feel alone most days, it's hard I get by,
I am used to sorrow, and these tears that I cry.
I am used to insensitivity, to daily rejection,
And now I have no more protection.
People are harsh they don't see me as ill,
They look down upon me when the tears start to spill.
They laugh at my heartache, they can not see,
But I guess that is part of this journey.
I am the brave one, I am strong,
If they had to endure this they probably couldn't go on.
I must have been chosen, I was picked out,
Although I never wanted this rout.
I must continue to move forward, keep moving on,
Although it's here for my life, it's made me strong.

God's Wounded Bird

I know that god made me different, he never had to speak a word.
I am special to him, I am god's wounded bird.
He protects me different looks after me with care, he knows my sufferings,
The burden he does share.
He carries me at my weakest, when I can no longer fly,
He lets me rest in his arms, and holds me when I cry.
He gave me this trial, because he knew I could get by,
He promised me a ticket to heaven, if I wait until my time to die.
He told me I must endure this heartache that it is my destiny,
And that I will have my place in paradise when he calls on me.
He told me it would make me stronger, although there would be days I would lag,
He told me I would have to keep going even though I'd drag.
He told me he would hold my hand, pick me up each time I'd fall,
He would keep pushing me, and help me endure it all.
Although there are days I want to give up I know he's by my side,
Guiding me, nurturing me, giving me the strength I am denied.
He does not always have to tell me I know that he is there,
I can sense his presence, sense his love, I know that he does care.
Although he made me different he never had to speak a word,
I am special to him, I am god's wounded bird.

In my poems of depression I did not want to live, but knowing I did not have a choice the only thing I could think to do was write it out. Those days were the hardest I ever had to live. And still live.

It would be so easy to give up. It is the most hopeless time nothing can make it better it just has to pass on its own. And trying to understand it and live with it has been the most challenging of all experiences. I don't know why I am a depressed person. But I know now that I don't need a reason. I am someone who had a good life. I know now that it is just the way my brain works and that is easier to accept now. I do not have to explain myself to others. I did not ask to be like this, I do not make myself feel this way, its just the way it is.

I hope this book has brought comfort to those out there that experience the same heartaches.
I felt that I should let my guard down and reach out and help those that are feeling lonely.
I always wished someone would reach out to me and let me know that they understand, that I am not really alone battling this illness.
I felt that this has been my purpose to possibly help those like me, or families of those like me. Maybe to help the world who is not familiar to ours to open there eyes and also reach out. If there was just one chance that I helped anyone out there than this illness is almost worth the heartache. Because if you can't reach out to a fellow human being in need, than what are we here for?
This book has been about acceptance, reaching out to others,
And coping with any form of mental illness, or any illness at all.
So I hope that I was able to reach out to at least one person and give them the strength to keep going.
I have felt for a long time that this was my purpose and I hope it helped someone in this world.
All I have ever wanted was understanding and acceptance.
That is what this book has offered.
It has been very scary to let my guard down and let everyone see my life for what it really is, not just the pretty picture I paint for them. But like I said even if I helped one person in this world to not feel alone than this book has been successful.
So thank you to all who have read it from the bottom of my heart.

ALTHOUGH THERE IS REALLY NO ENDING TO THIS BOOK SINCE IT IS A LIFE LONG ILLNESS AND BATTLE, I WILL CLOSE ON MY FAVORITE QOUTE OUT OF ONE OF MY POEMS:

"AND WHEN THE BURDEN GETS HEAVY AND YOU FEEL ALL HOPE IS LOST, JUST ONE MORE DAY TO LAUGH IS WORTH WHAT IT COST."

THE END,

BY CHRISTINA CHICKLOWSKI STAPLES